THE PREGNANCY BOOK

The Health Education

Authority's complete guide

to pregnancy, childbirth

and the first few weeks

with a new baby

Contents

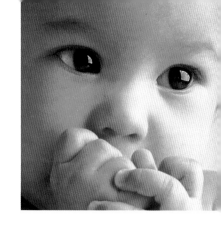

Your pregnancy at a glance

0-8 *weeks*

- Pregnancy test – you can have one from the first day of a missed period, if you wish (see **Finding out**, page 23).

- Make an early appointment to see your GP or a midwife if you know you're pregnant or think you may be (see **Finding out**, page 23). Begin to think about where you want your baby to be born (see **Deciding where to have your baby**, page 31). Ask about antenatal care (see **Antenatal care and antenatal classes**, page 47)

- Some mothers start to feel sick or tired around this time or have other minor physical problems for a few weeks (see **Common minor problems**, page 73).

- Try to eat a balanced diet (see pages 8-10).

8-12 *weeks*

- You'll probably attend your first antenatal appointment. Appointments will usually be monthly at first (see **Antenatal care and antenatal classes**, page 47).

- Ask about your rights at work and the benefits available (see **Rights and benefits**, page 126).

- If you're on Income Support or Income-based Jobseeker's Allowance, ask your doctor or midwife for form FW8 for milk tokens (see **Rights and benefits**, page 126)

- Make a dental appointment. Dental care is free during pregnancy.

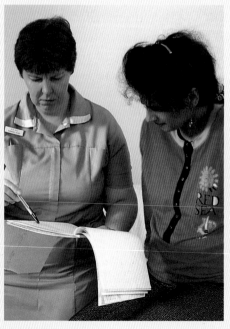

12-16 *weeks*

- Find out about antenatal classes if you have not already done so (see **Antenatal care and antenatal classes**, page 47).

- Begin to think about how you want to feed your baby (see **The feeding question**, page 63).

- Make sure you're wearing a bra which supports well.

- You may be offered an ultrasound scan which will show your baby moving. Your partner may like to see this too (see **Antenatal care and antenatal classes**, page 47).

- If you've been feeling sick and tired in the early weeks, you will probably start to feel better around this time.

- You may be offered tests to check for abnormalities in the baby (see pages 53-55).

16-20 *weeks*

- You *may* start to feel your baby move (see **How the baby develops**, page 25).

- Your tummy will begin to get bigger and you'll need looser clothes.

- You may feel a new surge of energy around this time.

- Try to do your pregnancy exercises regularly (see **Your health in pregnancy**, page 8). Ask your doctor or midwife to let you hear your baby's heartbeat.

20-24 *weeks*

- Your womb will begin to enlarge more rapidly and you'll really begin to look pregnant.

- You may feel hungrier than before. Stick to a sensible balanced diet (see **Your health in pregnancy**, page 8).

- Make sure you've booked into antenatal classes if you wish to attend (see pages 47-51).

24-28 *weeks*

- Get your maternity certificate, Form MAT B1, from your doctor or midwife (see **Rights and benefits**, page 126).

- If you're taking maternity leave, inform your employer in writing *at least* three weeks before you stop work (see **Rights and benefits**, page 126).

- If you're claiming Statutory Maternity Pay (SMP), write to your employer at least three weeks before you stop work (see **Rights and benefits**, page 126).

- If you're claiming Maternity Allowance, do so as soon as you can after you are 26 weeks pregnant (see **Rights and benefits**, page 126).

5

28-32 weeks

- If you're on Income Support, Income-based JobSeeker's Allowance or Family Credit, you can claim a lump sum maternity payment to help buy things for your new baby (see **Rights and benefits**, page 126).

- Think about what you need for the baby, if you have not already done so (see **What you need for the baby**, pages 81-84).

- If you have young children, spend time getting them used to the idea of a new baby.

- Check that your shoes are comfortable. If you get tired, try to rest with your feet above the level of your heart.

- You'll probably now attend for antenatal care every fortnight.

32-36 weeks

- Make arrangements for the birth, in hospital or at home. If you have children already, decide who will look after them.

- Pack your bag ready for the hospital, or make sure that you have been provided with a home delivery pack.

- You'll probably be attending antenatal classes now (see **Antenatal care and antenatal classes,** page 47).

- You may be more aware of your womb tightening from time to time. These are mild contractions (see **Labour and birth,** page 85).

- You may feel quite tired. Make sure you get plenty of rest.

36 weeks onwards

- You'll probably be attending antenatal care weekly until your baby is born.

- Make sure you have all important telephone numbers handy in case labour starts (see **Labour and birth,** page 85).

- The last few weeks can seem very long. Plan some interesting things to do to take your mind off waiting.

- Telephone your hospital or midwife if you have any worries about labour or the birth.

Introduction

Every parent is different, just as every baby is different. So there can't be many rules to having a baby. But you will find a lot of information in these pages which should help you to decide what you will do, how you will cope and, most of all, how you can best enjoy both pregnancy and your baby.

Chapter 1 is about what you can do to make sure you and your baby stay healthy during your pregnancy. The book then takes you through pregnancy, birth and the first two weeks of caring for your baby. You may want to read some chapters several times, or look up specific things which interest or concern you. To find a topic quickly, just look at the index at the back of the book.

If there is anything which puzzles you, or if you need further explanation, don't hesitate to ask your doctor, midwife or health visitor.

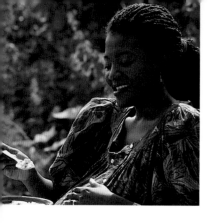

1 Your health in pregnancy

T his chapter describes some of the things you should think about to make sure you and your baby stay healthy during pregnancy.

WHAT SHOULD YOU EAT?

It's never too early for healthy eating. If you begin before you get pregnant you'll give your baby a flying start. Eating healthily during pregnancy will help your baby develop and grow and will keep you fit and well. You don't need to go on a special diet, but you need to make sure that you eat a mixture of different foods each day in order to get all the various nutrients that you and your baby need.

You'll also need to avoid certain foods during pregnancy to be on the safe side.

- **Eat plenty of fruit and vegetables** as these help to provide the vitamins and minerals you need, as well as fibre which helps digestion and prevents constipation. Eat them lightly cooked in a little water or raw to get the most out of them. Frozen and tinned fruit and vegetables are good too.

- **Starchy foods like bread, potatoes, rice, pasta and breakfast cereals** are an important part of any diet and should, with vegetables, form the main part of any meal. They are satisfying, without containing too many calories, and are an important source of vitamins and fibre. Try eating wholemeal bread and wholegrain cereals when you can.

- **Lean meat, fish, eggs, cheese, beans and lentils** are all good sources of nutrients. Eat some every day.

- **Dairy products, like milk, cheese and yoghurt** are important as they contain calcium and other nutrients needed for your baby's development. You can get milk free if you are on Income Support or Income-based Jobseeker's Allowance (see page 127).

- **Try to cut down on sugar and sugary foods** like sweets, biscuits and cakes and sugary drinks like cola. Sugar contains calories without providing any of the other nutrients the body needs. It also adds to the risk of tooth decay.

- **Cut down on fat and fatty foods as well.** Most of us eat far more fat than we need. Fat is very high in calories and too much increases the risk of heart disease. Avoid fried foods, trim the fat off meat, use spreads sparingly and go easy on foods like pastry, chocolate and chips which contain a lot of fat. Choose low-fat varieties of dairy products, for example semi-skimmed or skimmed milk, low-fat yoghurt and half-fat hard cheese.

VITAMINS AND MINERALS

- Green, leafy vegetables, lean meat, dried fruit and nuts★ (see page 10) contain **iron**. If you are short of iron you're likely to get very tired and may suffer from anaemia.

- Citrus fruit, tomatoes, broccoli, blackcurrants and potatoes are good sources of **vitamin C**, which you need to help you to absorb iron.

- Dairy products, fish with edible bones like sardines, bread, nuts★ (see page 10) and green vegetables are rich in **calcium**, which is vital for making bones and teeth.

- Margarine or oily fish (like tinned sardines) contain **vitamin D** to keep your bones healthy. The best source of vitamin D is sunlight, so try to get out for a while every day, but avoid sunburn by using high protection sunblock.

- You need extra **folic acid** from the time you start trying to conceive until the 12th week of pregnancy. This helps prevent spina bifida and other related conditions. You can get folic acid from green, leafy vegetables, but don't overcook them as this destroys the vitamin. Some breakfast cereals and breads have had folic acid added to them, so look at the label. You will also need to take a supplement of folic acid to make sure you're getting enough of this vitamin. Take a 400 microgram (0.4 milligram) folic acid tablet every day. These are available from pharmacies and supermarkets or your GP may be able to prescribe them for you. Ask your GP or pharmacist for advice.

VITAMIN SUPPLEMENTS

It's best to get the vitamins and minerals you need from the food you eat. Some people, like those on a restricted diet, need extra, especially vitamin D. Your doctor will tell you if you need vitamin supplements. Don't take extra vitamin A supplements without advice as too much could harm your baby.

FOLIC ACID

This vitamin is special. You need to take a 400 microgram (0.4 milligram) tablet every day from the time you start trying to conceive. Continue taking the supplement right up until you're 12 weeks pregnant. Even if you didn't take folic acid before conceiving, it's worth starting as soon as you find out that you're pregnant and you should still continue until you're 12 weeks pregnant. If you have had a baby with spina bifida before, have coeliac disease, or are taking medication for epilepsy, you will need to take a bigger dose of folic acid. Speak to your doctor about this.

Foods carrying this mark have added folic acid.

If you're on a restricted diet, e.g. gluten-free or vegan, talk to your doctor, who may refer you to a dietitian. You may find it helpful to have some extra advice on how to eat healthily during pregnancy.

Have drinks which contain caffeine – coffee, tea and colas – in moderation, as there may be a slight risk that too much caffeine will affect your baby's birthweight. Try decaffeinated tea and coffee, fruit juice or mineral water.

PREGNANCY AND WEIGHT

Most women gain between 10 –12.5kgs (22 – 28lbs). Weight gain varies a great deal and depends on your weight before pregnancy. If you're concerned, talk to your midwife or GP. They may have special advice for you if you weigh more than 100kg or under 50kg.

TAKE CARE WITH SOME FOODS

Besides eating a wide variety of foods, there are certain precautions you will need to take in order to safeguard your baby's well being as well as your own.

- **Cook all meat and poultry thoroughly** so that there is no trace of pink or blood and wash all surfaces and utensils after preparing raw meat. This will help to avoid infection with Toxoplasma, which may cause toxoplasmosis and can harm your baby (see page 16).

- **Wash fruit, vegetables and salads** to remove all traces of soil which may contain Toxoplasma.

- **Make sure eggs are thoroughly cooked** until the whites and yolks are solid, to prevent the risk of Salmonella food poisoning.

- **Avoid eating all types of paté and mould-ripened soft cheese**, like brie and camembert, and similar blue-veined varieties because of the risk of Listeria infection. Although this is a very rare disease, it is important to take special precautions during pregnancy because even the mild form of the illness can lead to miscarriage, stillbirth or severe illness in the newborn.

- **Drink only pasteurised or UHT** milk which have had the harmful germs destroyed. If only raw or green-top milk is available, boil it before you drink it. Don't drink unpasteurised goat's milk.

- **Don't eat liver or liver products**, like liver paté or liver sausage, as they may contain a lot of vitamin A. Too much vitamin A could harm your baby.

- **Avoid eating peanuts★ and foods containing peanut products** (e.g. peanut butter, **unrefined** groundnut oil, some snacks, etc.) if you or your baby's father or any previous children have a history of hayfever, asthma, eczema or other allergies. This may reduce the risk of your baby developing a potentially serious allergy to peanuts. Read food labels carefully and if you are still in doubt about the contents, avoid these foods.

FOR GENERAL HYGIENE

- Wash your hands before handling any food.

- Thoroughly wash all fruit and vegetables, including ready-prepared salads, before eating.

- Cook raw meat and poultry thoroughly and make sure that ready-to-eat poultry and cooked chilled meals are reheated thoroughly and are piping hot before they are eaten.

- Always wash your hands after handling raw meat or poultry and make sure that raw foods are stored separately from prepared foods. Otherwise there is a risk of contamination.

- Wear gloves and wash them and then your hands thoroughly after gardening or handling soil.

- Ask your doctor or clinic for a copy of *Enjoy healthy eating*, a free booklet published by the Health Education Authority, and also the free Department of Health leaflet, *While you are pregnant: how to avoid infection from food and from contact with animals.*

SMOKING

When you smoke, carbon monoxide and nicotine passes into your lungs and blood stream. This means that: a) your baby gets less oxygen and cannot grow as well as it should, and b) the nicotine makes your baby's heart beat faster. Constantly breathing in other people's smoke may also have a harmful effect.

IF YOU STOP SMOKING NOW:

- you're more likely to have a healthier pregnancy and a healthier baby;

- you'll cope better with the birth;

- your baby will cope better with any birth complication;

- your baby is less likely to be born too early and have to face the additional breathing, feeding and health problems which so often go with prematurity (see page 108);

- your baby is less likely to be born underweight and have extra problems in keeping warm. Babies of mothers who smoke are, on average, 200g (about 8 oz) lighter than other babies. These babies may have problems during and after labour and are more prone to infection;

- it will be better for your baby later too. Children whose parents smoke are more likely to suffer later on from illnesses which need hospital treatment (such as asthma);

- you will reduce the risk of cot death.

The sooner you stop, the better. But stopping even in the last few weeks of pregnancy can be beneficial. If any members of your household smoke, their smoke can affect you and the baby both before and after birth. They can help you and the baby by giving up now. Perhaps you could try to stop together.

SMOKING YOUR ACTION PLAN

Stop completely – it's never too late.

- ***Choose a day.*** *Will the first few days be easier during a working week or over a weekend? When you're busy or relaxed? Whatever you choose, stop completely on that day.*

- ***The day before.*** *Get everything ready; review your plan. Get rid of cigarettes.*

- ***Get help.*** *Ask friends for understanding and support. Consider asking your midwife, health visitor or practice nurse for advice.*

It might help to:

- *find something to do with your hands, like knitting;*

- *when you feel the urge to smoke, do something else instead – phone a friend, do some exercises, read, make a drink;*

- *reward yourself with the money you have saved.*

You may need extra help: read the free Health Education Authority booklet, Stopping smoking made easier, or phone Quitline on 0800 00 22 00 (0800 84 84 84 in Scotland; 0345 697500 in Wales), or the Ulster Cancer Foundation on 01232 663281 in Northern Ireland, for details of local support services.

1 UNIT =

½ pint ordinary strength beer, lager or cider

or

a single measure of spirit (whisky, gin, bacardi, vodka, etc.)

or   *a small glass of wine*

or   *a small glass of sherry*

or   *a measure of vermouth or aperitif*

ALCOHOL

There is no evidence that light or occasional drinking in pregnancy will harm your baby. But research shows that heavy or frequent drinking can seriously harm your baby's development. To be on the safe side, stop altogether or stick to no more than one or two 'units' of alcohol once or twice a week.

If you're with friends who are drinking:

- find a non–alcoholic drink you enjoy;

- if you drink alcohol, sip it slowly to make it last;

- if people try to pressure you into drinking, refuse politely but firmly;

- don't drink more than one or two units once or twice a week.

If you have difficulty cutting down, talk to your doctor or midwife. Confidential help and support is available from local counselling services (look in the telephone directory or contact Alcohol Concern). See page 136 for national agencies who can help.

These apply to the 25 ml measure used in most of England and Wales. In some places, pub measures are larger than this. In Northern Ireland, a pub measure is 35 ml or 1½ units. In Scotland, it can either be 35 ml or 25 ml. Home measures are usually more generous.

PILLS, MEDICINES AND OTHER DRUGS

HERBAL AND HOMEOPATHIC REMEDIES AND AROMATHERAPY

Not all 'natural' remedies are safe in pregnancy. Make sure that your practitioner is qualified (contact the Institute for Complementary Medicine, see page 136) and tell him or her that you are pregnant. Tell your midwife or doctor which remedies you are using.

Some pills and medicines can harm your baby's health so, to be on the safe side, you should:

- assume that all medicines are dangerous until a doctor or pharmacist can tell you they are safe;

- make sure your doctor or dentist knows you're pregnant before prescribing anything or giving you treatment;

- talk to your doctor at the first possible moment if you take regular medication.

But do remember that it is safer to take some medicines, for example those used to treat epilepsy and

diabetes, than to leave the illness untreated.

Drugs of addiction (street drugs) can harm your baby. Taking cocaine or smoking crack may be especially harmful because both cause a sudden drop in blood and oxygen to the placenta. It's important to talk to your doctor or midwife straight away so they can refer you to a maintenance reduction programme. For more information contact SCODA (the Standing Conference on Drug Abuse, see page 136), or the National Drugs Helpline on 0800 776600.

X-rays should be avoided in pregnancy if possible. Make sure your dentist knows you are pregnant.

PHYSICAL ACTIVITY

The more active and fit you are during pregnancy, the easier it will be for you to cope comfortably with your changing shape and weight gain. You are also more likely to have a normal labour and get back into shape after the birth. If you feel tense after a hard day's work, physical activity is an excellent way of relaxing and it will help you to sleep soundly.

Keep up your normal daily physical activity or exercise (sport, or dancing, or just walking to the shops and back) for as long as you feel comfortable. Don't exhaust yourself and remember that you may need to slow down as your pregnancy progresses, or if your doctor advises you to. If in doubt, consult your doctor or midwife.

- If you were inactive before you were pregnant, don't suddenly take up strenuous exercise. Start gently.

- Try to keep up regular exercise at least three times a week. If you can't manage that, any amount is better than nothing.

- If you take vigorous exercise, remember to start gradually and slow down comfortably.

- Avoid any strenuous exercise in hot weather.

- Drink plenty of fluids.

- If you go to exercise classes, make sure your teacher is properly qualified, and knows that you're pregnant and how far your pregnancy has progressed.

- You might like to try swimming because the water will support your increased weight. Some local swimming pools provide aquanatal classes with qualified instructors.

EXERCISES FOR A FITTER PREGNANCY

Every pregnant woman should try to fit these exercises into her daily routine. They will strengthen muscles to take a bigger load, make joints stronger and more flexible, improve circulation, ease backache and generally make you feel well.

Foot exercises can be done sitting or standing. They improve blood circulation, reduce swelling in the ankles, and prevent cramp in the calf muscles.

- Bend and stretch your foot vigorously up and down 30 times.

- Rotate your foot eight times one way and eight times the other way.

Pelvic rocking strengthens abdominal muscles and eases backache, which can be a problem in pregnancy. As your baby gets bigger you may find that the hollow in your lower back increases. This can give you backache.

- Standing with your feet hip-width apart and knees slightly bent, pull in your tummy and tilt your pelvis up. Now stretch up tall. You can also do pelvic rocking sitting on the edge of a chair, or on all fours:

- kneeling on all fours, hump up your back, draw in your abdominal muscles and look at your knees;

- now slowly relax your back (don't let it sag) and lift your head;

- do this slowly and rhythmically ten times, making your muscles work hard and moving your back carefully. Only move your back as far as you can comfortably.

Pelvic floor exercises help strengthen the muscles of the pelvic floor which come under great strain in pregnancy and childbirth. The pelvic floor consists of layers of muscles which stretch like a supportive hammock from the pubic bone (in front) to the end of the backbone. If your pelvic floor muscles are weak, you may find that you leak urine when you cough or sneeze. This is quite common and you needn't feel embarrassed. However, you can strengthen the muscles by doing the following exercise:

- close up your back passage as if trying to prevent a bowel movement;

- at the same time, draw in your vagina as if you are gripping a tampon, and your urethra as if to stop the flow of urine;

- hold for five seconds;

- repeat this exercise in sets of five, ten times a day.

Protect your back
- Sit up straight with your bottom against the back of your chair. Tuck a small cushion behind your waist if you wish.

- When you pick something up, bend your knees, not your back.

- Try to stand tall.

MEDICAL CHECKS

RUBELLA

Rubella (or German measles) can seriously affect your baby's sight and hearing and cause brain and heart defects in your baby if you catch it in the first four months of pregnancy. All children are now immunised against rubella at 12 to 15 months and again before they start school.

If you're not immune and you do come into contact with rubella, tell your doctor at once. Blood tests will show whether you have been infected, and you will then be better able to think about what action to take.

SEXUALLY TRANSMITTED INFECTIONS

Sexually transmitted infections (STIs) are very common and often there are no symptoms, so you may not know if you have one. However, many STIs can affect your baby's health during pregnancy and after birth. If you have any reason to believe that you or your partner could have an STI which was not diagnosed before pregnancy, you should go for a check-up as soon as you can. You can ask your GP or midwife or, if you prefer, go to a hospital clinic where you will also be guaranteed strict confidentiality. You can find your nearest clinic in your phone book, listed under the name of your health authority as genito-urinary medicine (GUM) clinic, or 'special' clinic, or the old name of Venereal disease (VD) clinic.

HUMAN IMMUNO-DEFICIENCY VIRUS (HIV) AND ACQUIRED IMMUNE DEFICIENCY SYNDROME (AIDS)

Current evidence suggests that an HIV positive mother in good health and without symptoms of the infection is unlikely to be adversely affected by pregnancy. However, 15% of children born to HIV positive mothers are likely to be infected. HIV positive mothers may also pass on the virus through breast milk. If you're HIV positive, talk to your doctor about your own health and the options open to you, or contact the organisations listed on page 136 for advice and counselling. It is possible to reduce the risk of transmitting HIV to your baby during pregnancy and after birth (see page 50).

If you suspect that you or your partner could be at risk of HIV, ask your doctor, midwife or health visitor, or go to a special clinic (see above) for advice before you decide whether or not to have a blood test for HIV. If you have a test, counselling should be offered afterwards to explain the result and the implications if it is either positive or negative.

HERPES

Herpes infection can be dangerous for the newborn baby. If you get recurring genital herpes, or if you or your partner develop any genital blisters or ulcers during your pregnancy, tell your doctor, midwife or obstetrician.

REMEMBER THAT YOU CAN GET INFECTED BY HIV IF YOU:

- *have intercourse, without using a condom, with anyone who is infected;*

- *use injectable drugs and share equipment with an infected person.*

CHICKEN POX

Catching chicken pox could be dangerous for your baby. If you've never had chicken pox and during your pregnancy you come into contact with a child or adult who has it, you should tell your doctor, midwife or obstetrician at once.

TOXOPLASMOSIS

This infection can damage your baby if you catch it during pregnancy, so take precautions (see page 10 and below). Some women have already had the infection before pregnancy and will be immune. If you feel you may have been at risk, discuss the matter with your GP, midwife or obstetrician. If you do catch toxoplasmosis while you are pregnant, treatment is available.

INHERITED CONDITIONS

Some diseases or conditions, like cystic fibrosis, haemophilia, muscular dystrophy, sickle cell disease and thalassaemia, are inherited from parents or grandparents. If you, your partner, or any relative has a condition which you know or suspect is inherited, or if you already have a baby with a disability, talk to your doctor about it. You may be able to have tests to check whether your baby is affected (see pages 50-51 and 53-55). Ask your GP to refer you to a genetic counsellor for specialist advice, if necessary, preferably before you conceive or in the early weeks of pregnancy.

ANIMALS

Cats' faeces may contain an organism which causes **toxoplasmosis** – a disease which can damage your baby. Avoid emptying cat litter trays while you're pregnant or, if no one else can do it, use disposable rubber gloves. Trays should be cleaned daily and filled with boiling water for five minutes.

Avoid close contact with sick cats and wear gloves when gardening – even if you don't have a cat – in case the soil is contaminated with faeces. Wash your hands and gloves after gardening. If you do come into contact with cat faeces, make sure you wash your hands thoroughly. Follow the general hygiene rules under **Take care with some foods** (page 10). For further information, contact the Toxoplasmosis Trust (see page 136).

Lambs and sheep can be a source of an organism called Chlamydia psittaci which is known to cause miscarriage in ewes. They also carry Toxoplasma. Avoid lambing or milking ewes and all contact with newborn lambs. If you experience flu–like symptoms after coming into contact with sheep, tell your doctor. Ask your doctor or clinic for a copy of the leaflet, *While you are pregnant: how to avoid infection from food and from contact with animals.*

WORK HAZARDS

If you work with chemicals, lead or X-rays, or in a job with a lot of lifting, you may be risking your health and the health of your baby. If you have any worries about this, you should talk to your doctor, midwife, occupational health nurse, your union representative or your personnel department.

If it is a known and recognised risk, it may be illegal for you to continue and your employer must offer you an alternative job, if one is available. If no job is available, your employer can dismiss you. However, this would not affect your rights to maternity pay and leave (see **Rights and benefits,** page 126).

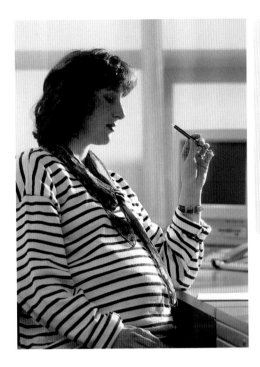

VDUs

Some women are concerned about reports of the effects of VDUs (visual display units on computer terminals and word processors) in pregnancy. The most recent research shows no evidence of a risk.

COPING AT WORK AND AT HOME

If you're at work during pregnancy you need to know your rights to antenatal care, leave and benefits which are set out on page 129. You may get extremely tired, particularly in the first and last weeks of your pregnancy. Try to use your lunch break to eat and rest, not to do the shopping. If travelling in rush hour is exhausting, ask your employer if you can work slightly different hours for a while.

Don't rush home and start another job cleaning and cooking. If possible, ask your partner to take over. If you're on your own, keep housework to a minimum, and go to bed early if you can.

SAFETY ON THE MOVE

*Road accidents are among the most common causes of injury in pregnant women. To protect both you and your unborn baby, **always** wear a seatbelt with the diagonal strap across your body between your breasts and the lap belt over your upper thighs. The straps should lie above and below your 'bump', not over it.*

2 Conception

To understand about conception and pregnancy, it helps to know about the male and female sexual organs. This information is useful in pregnancy too, when you want to ask questions and be clear about what you are told.

THE MAN'S SEXUAL ORGANS

Bladder

Vas deferens *This tube carries sperm from the testes to the prostate and other glands. These glands add secretions which are ejaculated along with the sperm.*

Urethra *The urethra is a tube running down the length of the penis from the bladder, through the prostate gland to an opening at the tip of the penis. Sperm travel down the urethra to be ejaculated.*

Penis *The penis is made of erectile tissue. This tissue acts like a sponge and, when it becomes filled with blood, the penis becomes hard and erect.*

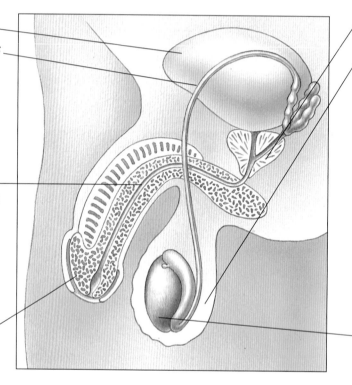

Prostate gland

Scrotum *This is the bag of skin which hangs outside the body and contains the testes. It helps to keep the testes at a constant temperature, just below the temperature of the rest of the body. This is necessary for sperm to be produced. In heat, the scrotum hangs down, away from the body, to keep the testes cool. When it is cold, the scrotum draws up closer to the body for warmth.*

Testes *There are two testes. These are where sperm are made.*

THE WOMAN'S SEXUAL ORGANS

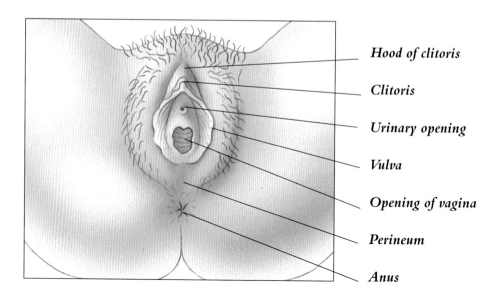

Hood of clitoris

Clitoris

Urinary opening

Vulva

Opening of vagina

Perineum

Anus

Fallopian tube

Ovary

Womb or uterus

Bladder

Cervix

Vagina

Urethra or water passage

Rectum

Anus

Perineum

Pelvis *The baby will pass through the pelvis when it is born.*

Womb or uterus *The womb is about the size and shape of a small upside down pear. It is made of muscle. It grows in size as the baby grows.*

Fallopian tubes *These lead from the ovaries to the womb.*

Ovaries *There are two ovaries, each about the size of an almond. They produce the eggs, or ova.*

Cervix *This is the neck of the womb. It is normally all but closed, with just a small opening through which blood passes during the monthly period.*

Vagina *The vagina is a tube about 8 cm (3 ins) long. It leads from the cervix down to the vulva, where it opens between the legs. The vagina is very elastic so it can easily stretch around a man's penis, or around a baby during labour.*

THE WOMAN'S MONTHLY CYCLE

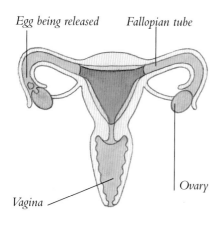

Egg being released   Fallopian tube

Vagina   Ovary

Egg progressing down the fallopian tube

Womb lining being shed

1. Each month a ripe egg or ovum (occasionally two) is released from one of the ovaries. This is called ovulation. The 'fingers' at the end of the fallopian tube help to direct the egg down into the tube. At the same time, the lining of the womb begins to thicken and the mucus in the cervix becomes thinner so that sperm can swim through it more easily.

2. The ripe egg begins to travel down the fallopian tube. It is here that it may be fertilised by a man's sperm if a couple have intercourse at this time. By now the lining of the womb is thick enough for the egg, if it is fertilised, to be implanted in it.

3. If the egg is not fertilised by a sperm, it passes out of the body through the vagina. It is so small that it cannot be seen. The lining of the womb is also shed in the monthly period of bleeding.

CONCEPTION

Egg

Sperm being ejaculated

Penis

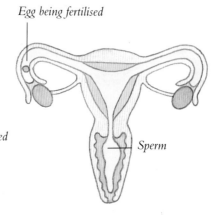

Egg being fertilised

Sperm

Attached embryo

1. A woman is most likely to conceive just after the time when she ovulates – when an egg has been released from one of her ovaries. During sexual intercourse, sperm are ejaculated from a man's penis into the woman's vagina. In one ejaculation, there may be more than 300 million sperm.

2. Most of the sperm leak out of the vagina again, but some begin to swim up through the cervix. At the time of ovulation the mucus in the cervix is thinner than usual to let the sperm pass through more easily. The sperm swim into the womb and so into the fallopian tube. One sperm may then join with the egg and fertilise it. Conception is said to have taken place.

3. During the week after fertilisation, the egg moves slowly down the fallopian tube and into the womb. It is already growing. The fertilised egg attaches itself firmly to the specially thickened womb lining. One ripe egg or ovum (occasionally two) is released from one of the woman's ovaries every month. It moves down into the fallopian tube where it may be fertilised by a man's sperm.

HORMONES

Hormones are chemicals which circulate in the blood of both men and women. They carry messages to different parts of the body, regulating certain activities and causing certain changes to take place. The female hormones, which include oestrogen and progesterone, control many of the events of the monthly cycle such as the release of the egg from the ovary and the thickening of the womb lining.

Once conception has occurred, the amount of oestrogen and progesterone increases. This causes the womb lining to build up, the blood supply to the womb and breasts to increase, and the muscles of the womb to relax to make room for the growing baby.

One ripe egg or ovum (occasionally two) is released from one of the woman's ovaries every month. It moves down into the fallopian tube where it may be fertilised by a man's sperm.

HEREDITY

Every normal human cell contains 46 chromosomes, except for the male sperm and female eggs. They contain 23 chromosomes each. When the sperm fuses with the egg and fertilisation takes place, the 23 chromosomes from the father pair with the 23 from the mother, making 46 in all.

The chromosomes are tiny thread-like structures which each carry about 2000 genes. It is the genes that determine the baby's inherited characteristics, such as hair and eye colour, blood group, height and build.

The fertilised egg contains one sex chromosome from the mother and one from the father. The sex chromosome from the mother's egg is always the same and is known as the X chromosome. But the sex chromosome from the father's sperm may be an X or a Y chromosome. If the egg is fertilised by a sperm containing an X chromosome, the baby will be a girl (XX). If the sperm contains a Y chromosome, then the baby will be a boy (XY).

A sperm is about 1/25th of a millimetre long and has a head, neck and tail. The tail moves from side to side so that the sperm can swim up the vagina into the womb and fallopian tubes.

THE BEST TIME TO GET PREGNAN'

An egg lives for about 12 to 24 hours after it is released from the ovary. If conception is to take place it must be fertilised within this time. Sperm can live for several days inside the woman's body. If you make love a day or so before ovulation, the sperm will have time to travel up the fallopian tubes and will be waiting when the egg is released. So the chances are highest if you make love on the day before ovulation (see chart).

Most women ovulate between 12–14 days before their next period.

Days | *First day of last period* | | | | | | Ovulation

| 27 | 28 | 1 | 2 | 3 | 4 | 5 | 6 | 7 | 8 | 9 | 10 | 11 | 12 | 13 | 14 | 15 | 16 | 17 | 18 | 19 | 20 | 21 | 22 | 23 | 24 | 25 | 26 | 27 | 28 |

*You are most likely to conceive
if you have intercourse
about this time.*

TWINS

Identical twins are the result of one fertilised egg splitting into two separate cells. Each cell grows into a baby. Because they originally came from the same cell, the babies have the same genes. They are the same sex and look very like each other. Non-identical twins are more common. They are the result of two eggs being fertilised by two sperm at the same time. The babies may not be the same sex and will probably look no more alike than other brothers and sisters.

Twins happen about once in every 80 pregnancies. A couple is more likely to have twins if there are twins in the woman's family. Triplets are much more rare and quads rarer still, although nowadays the use of drugs in the treatment of infertility has made multiple births more common. It is usually possible to find out if you are expecting twins by about the end of the second month of your pregnancy. An ultrasound scan is needed (see pages 52 and 53). It is a good idea to contact support groups like TAMBA (Twins and Multiple Births Association) and the Multiple Births Foundation (see page 135) before the babies are born.

FINDING OUT IF YOU'RE PREGNANT

THE SIGNS OF PREGNANCY

The earliest and most reliable sign of pregnancy, for women who have a regular monthly cycle, is a missed period. Sometimes women who are pregnant have a very light period, losing only a little blood. Other signs of pregnancy are listed below.

- **Feeling sick** – you may feel sick, or even be sick, not necessarily in the morning, but at any time.

- **Changes in your breasts** – often the breasts become larger and feel tender, rather as they may do before a period. They may tingle. The veins may show up more and the nipples may darken and stand out.

- **Needing to pass water more often.** You may find that you have to get up in the night to do so.

- **Being constipated.**

- **An increased vaginal discharge** without any soreness or irritation.

- **Feeling tired.**

- **Having a strange taste in your mouth** – many women describe it as metallic.

- **'Going off' certain things** like tea or coffee, tobacco smoke or fatty food, for example.

Some women don't even need these signs. They just 'know' that they are pregnant.

PREGNANCY TESTS

Pregnancy tests can be carried out on a sample of urine from the first day of a missed period – that is, about two weeks after conception. You can collect urine at any time of the day. Use a clean, soap-free, well-rinsed container to collect it. You may get pregnancy tests free from your GP or family planning clinic. Many pharmacists and most pregnancy advisory services also offer tests, usually for a small fee. You can also buy do-it-yourself pregnancy testing kits from pharmacists. They can be expensive but give you a quick result and you can do the test in private. Follow the instructions to be sure of a reliable result.

THE RESULTS OF THE TEST

A positive test result is almost certainly correct. A negative result is less reliable. You could wait a week and try again, or go straight to your doctor.

SEE YOUR DOCTOR

Whether or not you have had a pregnancy test, you should see your doctor as soon as you think you are pregnant. Being pregnant may affect your GP's treatment of any current or future illness. Your GP will also be able to advise you about antenatal care in your area and put you directly in touch with a midwife if you wish.

Information about the services available is given in the chapters on Deciding where to have your baby and Antenatal care and antenatal classes (see pages 31 and 47). It may help to look at these chapters before you talk to your doctor.

WORKING OUT WHEN YOUR BABY IS DUE

Use the chart below to work out your 'EDD' – expected date of delivery (or 'EDC' – expected date of confinement). Pick out the date of the first day of your last monthly period from the figures in black.

The date your baby is due is immediately underneath it in blue. For example, if your last period started on March 12, your baby will be due around December 17. Remember that this date is no more than a rough guide and it is based on a 28–day cycle.

January	1	2	3	4	5	6	7	8	9	10	11	12	13	14	15	16	17	18	19	20	21	22	23	24	25	26	27	28	29	30	31	**January**
October	8	9	10	11	12	13	14	15	16	17	18	19	20	21	22	23	24	25	26	27	28	29	30	31	1	2	3	4	5	6	7	November
February	1	2	3	4	5	6	7	8	9	10	11	12	13	14	15	16	17	18	19	20	21	22	23	24	25	26	27	28				**February**
November	8	9	10	11	12	13	14	15	16	17	18	19	20	21	22	23	24	25	26	27	28	29	30	1	2	3	4	5				December
March	1	2	3	4	5	6	7	8	9	10	11	12	13	14	15	16	17	18	19	20	21	22	23	24	25	26	27	28	29	30	31	**March**
December	6	7	8	9	10	11	12	13	14	15	16	17	18	19	20	21	22	23	24	25	26	27	28	29	30	31	1	2	3	4	5	January
April	1	2	3	4	5	6	7	8	9	10	11	12	13	14	15	16	17	18	19	20	21	22	23	24	25	26	27	28	29	30		**April**
January	6	7	8	9	10	11	12	13	14	15	16	17	18	19	20	21	22	23	24	25	26	27	28	29	30	31	1	2	3	4		February
May	1	2	3	4	5	6	7	8	9	10	11	12	13	14	15	16	17	18	19	20	21	22	23	24	25	26	27	28	29	30	31	**May**
February	5	6	7	8	9	10	11	12	13	14	15	16	17	18	19	20	21	22	23	24	25	26	27	28	1	2	3	4	5	6	7	March
June	1	2	3	4	5	6	7	8	9	10	11	12	13	14	15	16	17	18	19	20	21	22	23	24	25	26	27	28	29	30		**June**
March	8	9	10	11	12	13	14	15	16	17	18	19	20	21	22	23	24	25	26	27	28	29	30	31	1	2	3	4	5	6		April
July	1	2	3	4	5	6	7	8	9	10	11	12	13	14	15	16	17	18	19	20	21	22	23	24	25	26	27	28	29	30	31	**July**
April	8	9	10	11	12	13	14	15	16	17	18	19	20	21	22	23	24	25	26	27	28	29	30	31	1	2	3	4	5	6	7	May
August	1	2	3	4	5	6	7	8	9	10	11	12	13	14	15	16	17	18	19	20	21	22	23	24	25	26	27	28	29	30	31	**August**
May	8	9	10	11	12	13	14	15	16	17	18	19	20	21	22	23	24	25	26	27	28	29	30	31	1	2	3	4	5	6	7	June
September	1	2	3	4	5	6	7	8	9	10	11	12	13	14	15	16	17	18	19	20	21	22	23	24	25	26	27	28	29	30		**September**
June	8	9	10	11	12	13	14	15	16	17	18	19	20	21	22	23	24	25	26	27	28	29	30	1	2	3	4	5	6	7		July
October	1	2	3	4	5	6	7	8	9	10	11	12	13	14	15	16	17	18	19	20	21	22	23	24	25	26	27	28	29	30	31	**October**
July	8	9	10	11	12	13	14	15	16	17	18	19	20	21	22	23	24	25	26	27	28	29	30	31	1	2	3	4	5	6	7	August
November	1	2	3	4	5	6	7	8	9	10	11	12	13	14	15	16	17	18	19	20	21	22	23	24	25	26	27	28	29	30		**November**
August	8	9	10	11	12	13	14	15	16	17	18	19	20	21	22	23	24	25	26	27	28	29	30	31	1	2	3	4	5	6		September
December	1	2	3	4	5	6	7	8	9	10	11	12	13	14	15	16	17	18	19	20	21	22	23	24	25	26	27	28	29	30	31	**December**
September	8	9	10	11	12	13	14	15	16	17	18	19	20	21	22	23	24	25	26	27	28	29	30	31	1	2	3	4	5	6	7	October

KNOWING THAT YOU'RE PREGNANT

'I thought when I first got pregnant, "This is fantastic, it's really different, it's never happened to me before." '

'I wasn't very pleased at first. I was a bit shocked, I think, more than anything, and it took me about three months to get used to the idea that I was pregnant. I don't think I could believe it at first.'

You may feel very happy or excited when you discover that you are pregnant, but you shouldn't worry if you don't. Even if you have been looking forward to pregnancy, it is not unusual for your feelings to take you by surprise. And if your pregnancy was unplanned, then you may feel quite confused. Give yourself a little time to adjust to the idea of being pregnant. Even though you may feel rather anxious and uncertain now, this does not mean that you won't come to enjoy your pregnancy or to welcome the idea of the baby. Discuss your feelings with your midwife or doctor who will help you to adjust to your pregnancy, or in England, Scotland or Wales will give you advice if you are not happy to continue with it. You may want to share the news with family and friends immediately or wait a while until you've sorted out how you feel. But do begin to think about your antenatal care (that is, the care you'll receive leading up to the birth of your baby) and where you would like to have your baby. The earlier you begin to organise this, the more chance you will have of getting what you want.

3 How the baby develops

THE TIMING OF PREGNANCY

Doctors and midwives in the UK time pregnancy from the first day of a woman's last menstrual period, not from conception. So what is called 'four weeks pregnant' is actually about two weeks after conception. Pregnancy normally lasts for 37 to 42 weeks from the first day of your last period. The average is 40 weeks. If you're not sure about the date of your last period, then an ultrasound scan (see page 52) can give a good indication of when your baby will be due.

HOW THE BABY DEVELOPS

In the very early weeks, the developing baby is called an embryo. Then, from about eight weeks onward, it is called a fetus, meaning 'young one'.

WEEK 3

(Three weeks from the first day of your last menstrual period.) The fertilised egg moves slowly along the fallopian tube towards the womb. The egg begins as one single cell. This cell divides again and again. By the time the egg reaches the womb it has become a mass of over 100 cells, called an embryo, and is still growing. Once in the womb, the embryo burrows into the womb lining. This is called implantation.

Week 1

First day of your last menstrual period

Week 2

You conceive at about this time

Week 3

Week 4

At this point you will be called 4 weeks pregnant

Fertilised egg dividing and travelling down fallopian tube

Egg being fertilised

Egg being released from ovary

Ovary

Embryo implanting in womb lining

WEEKS 4–5

The embryo now settles into the womb lining. The outer cells reach out like roots to link with the mother's blood supply. The inner cells form into two and then later into three layers. Each of these layers will grow to be different parts of the baby's body. One layer becomes the brain and nervous system, the skin, eyes and ears. Another layer becomes the lungs, stomach and gut. The third layer becomes the heart, blood, muscles and bones.

The fifth week is the time of the first missed period when most women are only just beginning to think they may be pregnant. Yet already the baby's nervous system is starting to develop. A groove forms in the top layer of cells. The cells fold up and round to make a hollow tube called the neural tube. This will become the baby's brain and spinal cord, so the tube has a 'head end' and a 'tail end'. Defects in this tube are the cause of spina bifida.

At the same time the heart is forming and the baby already has some of its own blood vessels. A string of these blood vessels connects baby and mother and will become the umbilical cord.

WEEKS 6–7

There is now a large bulge where the heart is and a bump for the head because the brain is developing. The heart begins to beat and can be seen beating on an ultrasound scan.

Dimples on the side of the head will become the ears and there are thickenings where the eyes will be. On the body, bumps are forming which will become muscles and bones. And small swellings (called 'limb buds') show where the arms and legs are growing.

At seven weeks the embryo has grown to about 8mm long from head to bottom. (This measurement is called the 'crown–rump length'.)

WEEKS 8–9

A face is slowly forming. The eyes are more obvious and have some colour in them. There is a mouth, with a tongue.

There are now the beginnings of hands and feet, with ridges where te fingers and toes will be.

The major internal organs are all devloping – the heart, brain, lungs, kidneys, liver and gut.

At nine weeks, the baby has grown to about 17mm long from head to bottom.

The placenta
The placenta is rooted to the lining of the womb and separates the baby's circulation from the mother's. In the placenta, oxygen and food from the mother's bloodstream pass across into the baby's bloodstream and are carried to the baby along the umbilical cord. Antibodies, giving resistance to infection, pass to the baby in the same way, but so too can alcohol, nicotine and other drugs.

The umbilical cord
The umbilical cord is the baby's lifeline, the link between baby and mother. Blood circulates through the cord, carrying oxygen and food to the baby and carrying waste away again.

The amniotic sac
Inside the womb the baby floats in a bag of fluid called the amniotic sac. Before or during labour the sac, or 'membranes', break and the fluid drains out. This is called the 'waters breaking'.

WEEKS 10–14

Just 12 weeks after conception the fetus is fully formed. It has all its organs, muscles, limbs and bones, and its sex organs are well developed. From now on it has to grow and mature.

The baby is already moving about, but the movements cannot yet be felt.

By about 14 weeks, the heartbeat is strong and can be heard using an ultrasound detector. The heartbeat is very fast – about twice as fast as a normal adult's heartbeat.

At 14 weeks the baby is about 56mm long from head to bottom. The pregnancy may be just beginning to show, but this varies a lot from woman to woman.

ACTUAL SIZE
Week 14
At 14 weeks the baby is about 56 mm long from head to bottom. The pregnancy may be just beginning to show, although this varies a lot from woman to woman.

The lines on the skin of the fingers are now formed, so the baby already has its own individual fingerprint. Finger and toenails are growing and the baby has a firm hand grip.

At about 22 weeks, the baby becomes covered in a very fine, soft hair called 'lanugo'. The purpose of this isn't known, but it is thought that it may be to keep the baby at the right temperature. The lanugo disappears before birth, though sometimes just a little is left and disappears later.

At about 16 to 22 weeks you will feel your baby move for the first time. If this is your second baby, you may feel it earlier – at about 16 to 18 weeks after conception. At first you feel a fluttering or bubbling, or a very slight shifting movement, maybe a bit like indigestion. Later you can't mistake the movements and you can even see the baby kicking about. Often you can guess which bump is a hand or a foot and so on.

ACTUAL SIZE
Week 22
At 22 weeks, the head to bottom length is about 16cm.

WEEKS 15–22

The baby is now growing quickly. The body grows bigger so that the head and body are more in proportion and the baby doesn't look so top heavy. The face begins to look much more human and the hair is beginning to grow as well as eyebrows and eyelashes. The eyelids stay closed over the eyes.

WEEKS 23–30

The baby is now moving about vigorously and responds to touch and to sound. A very loud noise close by may make it jump and kick. It is also swallowing small amounts of the amniotic fluid in which it is floating and passing tiny amounts of urine back into the fluid. Sometimes the baby may get hiccups and you can feel the jerk of each hiccup. The baby may also begin to follow a pattern for waking and sleeping. Very often this is a different pattern from yours so, when you go to bed at night, the baby wakes up and starts kicking.

The baby's heartbeat can now be heard through a stethoscope. Your partner may even be able to hear it by putting an ear to your abdomen, but it can be difficult to find the right place. The baby is now covered in a white, greasy substance called 'vernix'. It is thought that this may be to protect the baby's skin as it floats in the amniotic fluid. The vernix mostly disappears before the birth.

At 24 weeks, the baby is called 'viable'. This means that the baby is now thought to have a chance of survival if born. Most babies born before this time cannot live because their lungs and other vital organs are not well enough developed. The care that can now be given in neonatal units means that more and more babies born early do survive.

At around 26 weeks the baby's eyelids open for the first time. The eyes are almost always blue or dark blue. It is not until some weeks after birth that the eyes become the colour they will stay, although some babies do have brown eyes at birth. The head to bottom length at 30 weeks is about 24 cm.

ACTUAL SIZE
Week 30
The head to bottom length at 30 weeks is about 24 cm

WEEKS 31–40

The baby is growing plumper so the skin, which was quite wrinkled before, is now smoother. Both the vernix and the lanugo begin to disappear.

By about 32 weeks the baby is usually lying downwards ready for birth. Some time before birth, the head may move down into the pelvis and is said to be 'engaged', but sometimes the baby's head does not engage until labour has started.

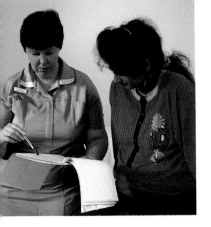

4 Deciding where to have your baby

The choice you have about where to have your baby and how you are cared for will depend to some extent on where you live. But what should be the same everywhere is that the care and the place should feel right for you.

SEE YOUR MIDWIFE OR DOCTOR AS SOON AS POSSIBLE IF:

- you are currently being treated for a chronic disease, such as diabetes or epilepsy;

- you are over 35, so that you can be offered additional tests for abnormalities in the baby;

- you are a teenager – there may be services available to you specifically for your age group;

- you have previously had a baby with spina bifida, Down's syndrome, or you have a family history of a genetic disorder such as cystic fibrosis or sickle cell disease – additional tests will be offered to you;

- you have previously had an ectopic pregnancy – you may be able to have an ultrasound scan to check that the pregnancy is in the womb.

It's important for you to make **informed** choices about the sort of care you would like and where you would like to give birth. Try to get information from as many sources as possible. You can go and look round the local hospital where there will probably be information leaflets about the services on offer. Midwives and your GP's surgery should also be able to tell you about the different options for care available in your area.

Don't hesitate to ask questions if you don't understand something or if you think that you need to know more. Midwives and doctors are there to help and support you. They want to make you feel as comfortable as possible with all aspects of the care you receive, both while you are pregnant and when you have your baby.

When you find out (or think) that you are pregnant, you can go either to your GP or direct to a midwife to discuss and arrange your care. Once you have found out what's available locally, talk things over with your GP or midwife. They will be able to offer you advice based on your

medical history and any previous pregnancies you may have had but, remember, the choice is yours. Don't forget, if you make your choice and then think that some other sort of care would be better for you and your baby, you can change your mind.

Your basic options will be to have your baby:

- in a **hospital** (a specialist unit with consultant obstetricians)

- at **home**

- in a **GP/midwife unit** (either as part of a large general hospital, in a smaller community hospital, or completely separate).

THE BASIC OPTIONS

Spend some time thinking about the following options. Discuss them before you come to a decision.

IN HOSPITAL

For the last 30 years most babies have been born in hospital. Many hospitals have tried hard to meet parents' wishes and to make labour and delivery as private and special as possible. All over the country maternity care staff are working even harder to make sure that women get kind, sympathetic and sensitive care. Hospital maternity units should become friendlier, more comfortable places, where you will be able to get to know the people who are caring for you. You will probably be asked many questions about your wishes so you should feel more in control over what's happening to you.

If there is more than one hospital in your district, and you can choose which to go to, try to find out about the practice in each so that you can decide which will suit you best. **Team midwifery** may be in operation which means that you will see a midwife from the same team each time you visit the hospital, including at the delivery of your baby. Or there may be a **Domino Scheme** which means that your midwife will attend you at home in labour, accompany you to hospital to deliver your baby, and then accompany you home after the delivery (usually six hours later). Midwifery care will then continue to be provided as necessary for 10 to 28 days.

Use the checklist on page 33 as a guide to the sort of questions to ask. Talk to your doctor or midwife. It's also a good idea to talk to other mothers who have recently had babies and ask them about their

experiences at local hospitals. You can contact other mothers through your local branch of the National Childbirth Trust, your local Community Health Council and AIMS (the Association for Improvements in the Maternity Services, see page 134).

AT HOME

Some women want to have their babies at home because:

- they feel they will be happier and better able to cope in a place they know and with their family around them;

- if they have other young children, there will be no need to leave them to go into hospital;

- they will have more privacy;

- they will be able to relax more and will not have to fit into a hospital routine;

- they are more likely to get to know the midwife who will be with them during the delivery.

One or two midwives will stay with you while you're in labour and, if any help is needed, will summon a doctor or send for an ambulance to get to the hospital in an emergency.

HOW TO BOOK IN FOR A HOSPITAL DELIVERY

Your GP or midwife will either send a letter to the hospital or give you one to take there. This is best done as early in your pregnancy as possible.

Ask your GP or midwife for the Department of Health's leaflet, How to get the best from maternity services.

31

HOW TO ARRANGE FOR A HOME DELIVERY

If you are considering a home delivery, first talk to your midwife and GP. Some people think that women should not have home births because they argue that they are unsafe. In fact, research suggests that a home delivery is as safe as a hospital delivery for women who have uncomplicated pregnancies. You have the right to choose to have your baby at home. Your doctor or midwife may advise against this if they think that you are at risk of complications during labour. However, this may be difficult to judge if this is your first baby.

Find out whether your own GP will be prepared to care for you during your pregnancy and a home delivery. If he or she cannot help, there may be another in the district who can. You can then register with this GP just for your maternity care and continue to see your own GP for any other medical treatment. The local supervisor of midwives (see box) or Local Health Authority (see page 134) can give you the names of GPs with a special interest in pregnancy and childbirth.

Alternatively, it is possible to arrange for maternity care to be led by a team of midwives. Contact the local supervisor of midwives at your nearest hospital who will

arrange for a midwife to visit you at home to discuss home delivery. The midwife may also be able to provide most or all of your antenatal care at home. You can contact her directly when labour starts and she will stay with you during labour and the birth of your baby.

IN A GP/MIDWIFE UNIT

This may be part of the hospital's ordinary maternity wards or a separate unit. Your baby can be delivered here by your community midwife, who has been involved in your antenatal care, and your GP (or sometimes by a hospital midwife). Some areas operate a **team midwifery** system (see page 31), so you may get to know who will deliver your baby.

Care in a GP/midwife unit can be more personal since you will usually be looked after by people you know. If the unit is part of the main hospital, then emergency facilities are there, should an unforeseen problem arise. This type of unit is generally used for women who are likely to have a normal delivery. The length of time you will remain in the unit after the birth depends on how well you and your baby are.

*Before you try to get answers to your questions and make your decision, it will help to read the chapter on **Labour and birth** (page 85).*

Deciding where to have your baby

THESE ARE THE KINDS OF QUESTIONS YOU MAY WISH TO ASK ABOUT A HOSPITAL:

Would you go to the hospital antenatal clinic for all or just some of your antenatal care appointments?

Does the antenatal clinic run an appointments system?

Does the hospital run antenatal classes?

Does the hospital offer team midwifery care or the Domino Scheme for delivery (see page 31)?

Will I be shown round the labour and postnatal wards before the birth?

Is there a chance for me to discuss and work out a birth plan?

Can I be seen by a woman doctor if I prefer?

ABOUT LABOUR AND DELIVERY:

Are fathers, close relatives or friends welcome in the delivery room?

Are they ever asked to leave the room, and why?

Does the hospital encourage women to move around in labour and find their own position for the birth, if that is what they want?

What is the hospital policy on induction, pain relief, routine monitoring, or any other aspect of labour that concerns you?

AFTERWARDS:

Are babies usually put to their mother's breast immediately after birth?

What services are provided for sick babies?

Are babies with their mothers all the time or is there a separate nursery?

Will the hospital encourage (and help) me to feed my baby 'on demand' if this is what I want to do?

Who will help me breastfeed my baby?

What is the normal length of stay?

What are visiting hours?

Are there any special rules about visiting?

BIRTH PLAN

A birth plan is a record of what you would like to happen during your labour and after the birth. You may be given an opportunity to draw up a birth plan during your antenatal care. If not, ask your midwife if you can do so. Discussing a birth plan with your midwife, preferably over several meetings, will give you the chance to ask questions and find out more information. It also gives the midwife the chance to get to know you better and understand your feelings and priorities. You will probably want to think about or discuss some points more fully with your partner, or friends and relatives, before reaching a decision. And you can, of course, change your mind at any time.

BREASTFEEDING

If you have decided to breastfeed, your birth plan should note that you want to put your baby to your breast straight after birth. This helps to get breastfeeding started. It should also note that you do not want your baby to be given any extra formula milk feeds, as this can hinder successful breastfeeding.

There is no one, correct way to give birth. All birth plans have to be drawn up individually and then discussed with your midwife. They depend not only on your own wishes, but also on your medical history and your own circumstances, and on what is available at your own hospital or unit. What may be safe and practical for one mother may not be a good idea for another.

You may be given a special form for a birth plan, or there may be room in your notes. You could use page 35 of this book. It's a good idea for you to keep a copy of your birth plan with you. The midwife or doctor who cares for you during labour will discuss it with you so they know your wishes. But remember, you may need to be flexible if complications arise with you or the baby. The doctor or midwife will tell you what they advise in your particular circumstances. Don't hesitate to ask questions if you need to.

Read the chapters on **Labour and birth** (page 85) and **The first few days with your new baby** (page 103) before talking to your midwife, to see if there is anything you feel strongly about and might wish to include. You may find it useful to think about some of these things. You may want to take this book with you to discuss with your midwife.

...and if you need any more information...

BIRTH PLAN

BIRTH PLAN

Do you want your partner, or a chosen companion(s), to be with you during labour?

....

Do you want your partner or companion to be with you if you have a Caesarean section or forceps delivery, for example?

....

Is equipment such as mats, a birthing chair or beanbags available to you if you want it, or can you bring your own?

....

Are there special facilities, like special rooms or birthing pools?

....

How do you want your baby's heart monitored if everything is straightforward?

....

Do you prefer to be cared for and delivered by women only?

....

Is it important for you to be able to move around when you're in labour?

....

What position would you like to be in for the birth?

....

If you think you would like pain relief, which sort do you want to try (see pages 87-89)? If you want to try to manage without pain relief, it's a good idea to note this in the birth plan too.

....

Are epidurals available at all times should you want one?

....

Are there other means, such as warm baths, massage or other therapies, that you would like to use to help you cope with labour?

....

What do you feel about an episiotomy?

....

Do you want your baby delivered straight on to your tummy or do you want your baby cleaned first?

....

Do you have any feelings about the injection usually given to you after the birth to help the womb contract?

....

How do you wish to feed your baby?

....

Do you want your baby close to you all the time? If you intend to breastfeed you should make a note that you want your baby close by you all the time or brought to you when hungry so that you can feed on demand.

....

Do you want your baby to have vitamin K, and by which route (see page 106)?

....

Is there anything you feel you may need extra help with?

....

Do you mind if students are present?

....

Do you need an interpreter?

....

Do you need a sign language interpreter?

....

Do you need a special diet?

....

Do you or your partner or companion have special needs that should be considered, for example, do you or your partner normally use a guide dog or a wheelchair?

....

Are there special religious customs you wish to be observed?

....

5 Feelings and relationships

From the minute you know you're pregnant, things begin to change. Your feelings change – feelings about yourself, about the baby, about your future. Your relationships change – with your partner, and also with parents and friends.

But you're still yourself, and you still have to get on with your life, whether pregnant or not. For this reason, adjusting to the changes that pregnancy brings isn't always easy. This chapter is about some of the worries that may crop up in pregnancy and some suggestions on how to handle them. But, of course, what may be a problem for one person may not be a problem for another. And what is helpful advice for some people may not be right for you. So take from these pages what you find useful, and don't bother about the rest.

'I think you have more extremes of emotion. You get more easily upset about things, and you can more easily get very happy about things.'

FEELINGS

'It frightens me, wondering what I've got to go through. People say different things, you know, so you don't know what to think.'

When you're pregnant it can sometimes seem as though you are not allowed to have other feelings as well. People expect you to be looking forward to the baby, to be excited and to 'bloom' all the time. You, yourself, may think that this is the way you ought to be. In fact, just like any other nine months in your life, you're likely to have times when you feel low. And pregnancy does bring extra reasons for feeling worried or down, just as it brings many reasons for happiness.

Hormonal changes taking place in your body are responsible for much of the tiredness and nausea that some women feel in the early months and for some of the emotional upsets which can happen. You may find you cry more easily, lose your temper more, and so on.

'I think it's a lot to do with mind over matter. I think the thing to do is just try and relax and not be frightened. I mean, it's happened to thousands and millions of people before you.'

Of course, there are many other reasons why you may feel rather down. You may have money worries or worries about work or where you are going to live. You may be anxious about whether you will cope as a parent, or about whether you're really ready to be a parent at all. And many of these anxieties may be shared by your partner or family as well.

Talking about your feelings to your partner, or to someone who is close to you, is often a relief and can help you get things in proportion. It may help your partner too. Making sure you keep yourself well and get plenty of sleep will also help.

Anyone who is tired and run down is likely to feel rather low, whether they are pregnant or not. And don't let the pregnancy take over your life. Keep on doing the things you enjoy. Although it's normal to have some worries while you are pregnant and to feel a bit down from time to time, it's a real cause for concern if you're feeling depressed for most of the time. Whatever the reason for your unhappiness, or even if there doesn't seem to be any reason at all, explain how you feel to your doctor, midwife or health visitor. Make sure they understand that you're talking about something more than just feeling low.

'I've enjoyed it. I've enjoyed the newness of it. I've enjoyed thinking of the baby. The only thing I haven't enjoyed is getting so big.'

'I loved every minute of being pregnant and went through a wonderful experience with labour.'

'Antenatal classes really helped. I met lots of women there who had the same fears as me. The midwife made us more confident by telling us what happens in labour. I felt well prepared.'

WORRYING ABOUT THE BIRTH

One worry that a lot of women have in pregnancy is whether labour and birth will be painful and how they will cope. It is difficult to imagine what a contraction might be like and no one can tell you – though many will try. However, factual information about the options open to you can help you to feel more confident and more in control.

Begin by reading the chapter on **Labour and birth** (page 85) with your partner, or a friend or relative who will be with you for the birth, if possible. Ask your midwife or doctor for any further information. Antenatal classes will also help to prepare you for labour and the birth (see pages 60–61).

Think about the sort of labour and birth you would like to have. You will probably have an opportunity to discuss this in more detail with your midwife and to draw up a birth plan during the later months of pregnancy (see page 35).

Talk to your partner too, or to someone close to you, and particularly to the person who will be with you in labour. Remember they may be anxious also. Together you can then work out ways in which to cope.

but how will I know if I'm in labour?

WORRYING ABOUT ABNORMALITY

'I want to know if it's alright. I think that's always at the back of your mind – you don't know whether it's alright. It's a worry that's always there.'

'I feel guilty at times. It's not just worrying about what you do and whether it will damage the baby. Sometimes I feel I just haven't thought about the baby, cared about it enough. I ought to be loving it more.'

'You hear such a lot and read such a lot in the newspapers about spina bifida and backward children and all that. You can't help but wonder about your own.'

'Now that I've felt it move and I've heard the heartbeat, I feel happier. Early on we worried much more.'

Everyone worries at some time that there may be something wrong with their baby. Some people find that talking openly about their fears helps them to cope. Others prefer not to dwell on the possibility of something being wrong.

Some women continue to worry because they are convinced that if something does go wrong it will be their fault. But while you can increase your baby's chances of being born healthy by eating well and by not smoking for example (see pages 8–11), you cannot cut out the risk entirely. There are certain problems which cannot be prevented, either because the causes are not known or because they are beyond anyone's control.

It may reassure you to know that 97% of babies born in the UK are normal, although some of these may have birthmarks or some other small variations. A further 1% of babies will be born with abnormalities that can be partly or completely corrected. About 2%, however, will suffer from some more severe disability. Regular antenatal care and careful observation during labour help so that action can be taken if necessary.

If you are particularly concerned, perhaps because someone in your family has a disability, or because someone you know has had a difficult birth, or even if you just feel very anxious, talk to your doctor or midwife as soon as possible. They may be able to reassure you or

offer you helpful information about tests which can be done in pregnancy (see pages 53-55).

COUPLES

Pregnancy is bound to bring about some quite big changes in a couple's relationship, especially if this is your first baby. For some people these changes happen easily, others find it harder to change. Everybody is different.

It's quite common for couples to find themselves having arguments every now and then during pregnancy, however much they are looking forward to the baby. Some of these may be nothing to do with the pregnancy, but others may be caused by one or other partner feeling worried about the future and how they are going to cope. Perhaps the most important thing to realise is that during pregnancy there are understandable reasons for the odd difficulty between you and also good reasons for feeling closer and more loving.

One practical question you will need to discuss is how you will cope with labour and whether your partner will be there. Many fathers do want to be present at their baby's birth. The chapter on **Labour and birth** (page 85) gives some suggestions on ways in which fathers can help and what it can mean to them to share this experience.

SEX IN PREGNANCY

Many people worry about whether it is safe to have sex during pregnancy. There is no physical reason why you shouldn't continue to have sexual intercourse right through a normal pregnancy, if you wish. It doesn't harm the baby because the penis cannot penetrate beyond the vagina. The muscles of the cervix and a plug of mucus, specially formed in pregnancy, seal off the womb completely.

Later in pregnancy, an orgasm, or even sexual intercourse itself, can set off contractions (known as Braxton Hicks' contractions, see page 86). You will feel the muscles of your womb go hard. There is no need for alarm as this is perfectly normal. If it feels uncomfortable, try your relaxation techniques or just lie quietly till the contractions pass.

If you have had a previous miscarriage, ask your doctor or midwife for advice. Your doctor or midwife will probably advise you to avoid intercourse if you have had heavy bleeding in pregnancy, and you should definitely not have intercourse once the waters have broken (see page 86) since this risks infection in the baby.

While sex is safe for most couples in pregnancy, it may not be all that easy. You will probably need to find different positions. This can be a time to explore and experiment together. The man on top can become very uncomfortable for the woman quite early in pregnancy, not just because of the baby, but because of tender breasts as well. It can also be uncomfortable if the man's penis penetrates too deeply. So it may be better to lie on your sides, either facing or with the man behind. Many couples find that a position in which the woman is on top is most comfortable.

Some couples find making love extra enjoyable during pregnancy while others simply feel that they don't want to have intercourse and prefer to find other ways of being loving or of making love. It's important to talk about your feelings to each other.

'You've got a bond between you. It's something that belongs to both of you.'

'Sometimes it draws us together and sometimes it sets us apart. When we first found out about the baby, we were on edge. We snapped at each other a lot. Then it got better. We really wanted each other and we were really looking forward to the baby coming. It's up and down.'

FAMILIES AND FRIENDS

'There's the feeling that you're being looked after. Not just by your husband and your parents and the hospital, but by your friends, by everybody. They're there behind you. I suppose they're wrapping me up in cotton wool, but it's still a nice feeling.'

' My mother starts telling me 'You must have this for the baby, you must have that', and trying to tell me what I should do. And bringing things like nappy pins and saying 'I didn't think you'd remember to get them.' It's irritating.'

'We seem to have got a lot closer. We often sit and talk and my mum remembers when I was tiny.'

'It's no good listening to other people. They only tell you about what happened to them. They tell you the bad parts too, not the good.'

In some ways pregnancy is very private, just to do with you and your partner, but there may be a lot of people around you who are also interested and concerned about your baby – parents, sisters, brothers and friends.

People can offer a great deal of help in all sorts of ways and you will probably be very glad of their interest and their support. But sometimes it can feel as if you're being taken over. If so, it can help everyone if you explain gently that there are some decisions that only you can take and some things that you prefer to do on your own. You may also find that being pregnant puts you on the receiving end of a lot of advice, and perhaps a bit of criticism too. Sometimes the advice is helpful, sometimes not. Sometimes the criticism can really hurt. The important thing is to decide what is right for you. After all, it is your pregnancy and your baby.

WORK

If you enjoy your work and the company of those you work with, you may have rather mixed feelings when the time comes to stop work before your baby is born. Try to make the most of these few weeks to enjoy doing the things you want to do at your own pace. It is also a good opportunity to make some new friends. You may meet other mothers at your antenatal classes (see pages 60-61) or you may get to know more people living close by, now that you have more time to stop and chat.

You may have decided that you are going to spend some time at home with your baby or you may be planning to return to work, either full or part-time, fairly soon after the birth. If you know that you will be going back to work, or even if you think you might be, you will need to start thinking about who will look after your baby well in advance. It is not always easy to find a satisfactory childcare arrangement and it may take you some time.

Any decision you make about childcare will be determined both by your income and the kind of facilities available locally. You may be lucky enough to have a relative willing to provide care. If not, you should contact your council social services department (in Northern Ireland your local Health and Social Services Trust) for a list of registered childminders and nurseries. Few nurseries take babies and prices are usually high. You may also want to consider organising care in your own home, either on your own or sharing with other parents.

Care in your own home does not need to be registered but you should satisfy yourself that your carer is experienced and trained to care for babies. Contact the National Childminding Association or Working for Childcare (see page 136) for more information.

COPING ALONE

'The baby's dad has gone. He wanted the baby at first but when things started to happen he didn't like it, so he's gone. But my mum has been to all my antenatal classes with me and everything, so she knows what's going on.'

'Sometimes I feel really low and think, "Oh God, I'm only 18 and it's for the rest of my life. Every time I go out I've got to get a baby sitter and things.'

'I talked to the hospital social worker about things and she told me all about managing on my own.'

If you're pregnant and on your own it's even more important that there are people with whom you can share your feelings and who can offer you support. Sorting out problems, whether personal or medical, is often difficult when you are by yourself and it's better to find someone to talk to rather than to let things get you down.

You may find it encouraging to meet other mothers who have also gone through pregnancy on their own. Gingerbread (see page 135) is a self-help organisation for one-parent families which has a network of local groups and can offer you information and advice. They will be able to put you in touch with other mothers in a similar situation if you wish.

If money is an immediate concern, read **Rights and benefits** (page 126) for information on what you can claim and your employment rights. Your local social security office, the DSS Freeline or local Citizens Advice Bureau (CAB) will be able to give you more advice. If you have housing problems, contact your local CAB or your local housing advice centre. Ask for the address from your local authority at the town hall.

The National Council for One Parent Families can also supply information on a range of topics from benefits to maintenance (see page 135). There may be a local support group in your area. Ask your health visitor.

Don't feel that, just because you don't have a partner, you have to go to antenatal visits and cope with labour on your own. You have as much right as anyone else to be accompanied by the person you choose – a friend, sister, or perhaps your mother. Involve your 'labour partner' in birth classes if you can and let him or her know what you want from them. There may be antenatal classes in your area run especially for single women. Ask your midwife.

Think about how you will manage after the birth. Will there be people around to help and support? If there is no one who can give you support it might help to discuss your situation with a social worker. Your doctor or hospital can refer you or you can contact the social services department of your local council directly.

If you're considering adoption or fostering you should discuss this with a social worker.

6 Mainly for men

Some pregnancies have been planned for months or years, but many are unexpected. Either way, you'll probably feel pretty mixed up. A baby means new responsibilities which, whatever your age, you may feel unready for.

YOUR FEELINGS ABOUT PREGNANCY

Your partner may have similar feelings. It's normal for both of you to feel like this. Your first pregnancy is a very important event. It will change your life and change can be frightening even if it's something you've been looking forward to. Money problems may be nagging at you – the loss of an income for a while, extra expenses for the baby and, if your partner returns to work, the cost of childcare. You may be worrying that your home isn't right or that you'll feel obliged to stay in a job you don't like. (It might help to look at the **Rights and benefits** section on page 126 and start planning ahead.)

Some men feel left out. Your partner's attention will be on what's happening inside her and she may want you to pay a lot more attention to her needs than usual. You may not have realised how much you relied on her to make you feel cared for and now that her attention is elsewhere you may feel quite lonely. Your loneliness may be increased if your partner doesn't want to make love, although some women find sex more enjoyable than ever. It varies from person to person. There's usually no medical reason to avoid sex but keep in mind:

- her breasts in the early weeks may be extremely painful;

- if there's any bleeding or pain avoid intercourse (and consult your doctor);

- make sure your partner is comfortable – you may need to try different positions as the pregnancy progresses.

If she's not interested in sex, try to find other ways of being close, but do talk about it. If she feels that you're trying to persuade her to do something she doesn't want, she may withdraw completely leaving both of you lonely.

Some men find it hard to make love during pregnancy. They feel strange doing it with 'someone else there' or may find their partner's changing shape disturbing. This is one situation when it helps to be careful what you say. Your partner may well feel uneasy about her changing body and may be very hurt if she thinks that you don't like it either.

' When the test was positive, I felt really excited, on a real high. We couldn't wait to tell everyone.'

(A FATHER)

'It was a shock at first, but now I'm getting used to the idea. We didn't plan it, but there's no problem with that. If it had been three years ago, when we first started living together, obviously it would have been a lot worse financially. That's the main factor.'

(A FATHER)

43

TALK ABOUT IT

'She became very absorbed in her own body, separate. I felt lonely and frightened of not doing the right thing.'

(A FATHER)

'My worries are to do with making sure that she's happy and comfortable and that.'

(A FATHER)

Confide in friends who are already fathers and will know what you're going through. You may want to protect your partner from your worries but she will almost certainly sense your concern. The more you keep it to yourself, the more she'll feel that you're moving away from her – just when she badly needs you to be there. If you're giving her the support she needs, then there's no need to leave your feelings out of the picture.

PHYSICAL FEELINGS

Believe it or not, men can get symptoms of pregnancy too! The most commonly reported ones are sleeplessness, indigestion and nausea. They are probably caused by stress, but are no less uncomfortable for that.

SUPPORTING YOUR PARTNER

'My wife one day couldn't stand the smell of me. I tried every different kind of soap, but it made no difference. In the end I asked the doctor about it.'

(A FATHER)

'I am happy to be involved. I want to know what she has to do. I like to feel involved, contributing to this, not just starting it.'

(A FATHER)

Something amazing is happening inside your partner's body. The closer you can get to her, the more you'll be able to share this experience. But at times closeness will seem impossible.

In the early weeks she may be prickly and irritable about the slightest things. Certain smells and tastes may make her nauseous. She may want only to sleep.

In the middle months you'll probably find that much of her energy returns and she may resent being treated 'like china'.

Towards the end the weight of the baby may drag her down. The tiredness and irritability of the early weeks often returns and she may start feeling quite frightened of the birth and be lonely without the company of friends at work.

If your partner is anxious, encourage her to talk about it. Many women are more used to listening than being listened to, so it may take a while before she feels able to open up. Be patient – the better you can learn to support each other now, the stronger your relationship will be when the baby arrives.

PRACTICAL SUPPORT

Your partner may be used to doing most of the housework as well as going out to work. If she continues to do all this work she'll tire herself out. Now is the time to start sharing the housework if you don't already do so. There are two areas where you can really help:

- cooking – in the early months the smell may put her off and if you cook she's more likely to eat what she needs;

- carrying heavy shopping can put a lot of strain on her back, so try to do the shopping yourself or together.

A FRIEND IN NEED

Pregnancy can be frightening so it will help if she knows that she's not alone. Start by reading the rest of this book with her so that you're both well informed. Some of the basic health advice is just as important for you as it is for her.

- Good eating is much easier if you're doing it together, so read pages 8-10 and start picking up the food habits you'll want to pass on to your child.

- Cigarette smoke is dangerous for babies. If you are a smoker read page 11 on how to stop.

- If you continue to smoke, don't smoke near your partner, don't offer her cigarettes and don't leave your cigarettes lying around.

- Go with her to the doctor if she's worried, or be sure to talk it through when she gets home.

- Be there if she has a scan (see page 52) and see your baby on the screen.

- If she needs to have extra tests (see pages 53-55) your support is especially important.

- Find out about antenatal classes for couples, or fathers' evenings at the hospital (see pages 60-61). The more you know about labour, the more you'll be able to help.

- Most men stay with their partners during labour but it's important that you're both happy about it. If you prefer not to be present, talk to your partner. You may be able to think of a friend or relative who could accompany her instead.

- Talk about what you both expect in labour (see page 34).

- Talk about the birth plan (see page 35). Fill it in together so you know what she wants and how you can help her achieve it. Support her if she changes her mind during labour. Be flexible.

- During labour she'll be far too involved with what's happening inside to pay much attention to the people around her. You can be her guide and interpreter.

PATERNITY LEAVE

Speak to your Human Resources department or your boss about the paternity leave entitlement in your company. More employers are now realising that partners need time off work when they have a new baby.

THE BIRTH – BEING PREPARED

A checklist for the final weeks

- *Make sure your partner can contact you at all times.*

- *Decide how you'll get to the hospital (if you're having a hospital birth).*

- *If you're using your own car, make sure it works and do a trial run to see how long it takes.*

- *Remember to pack a bag for yourself including snacks, a camera and film, and change for the telephone.*

'From time to time I became angry. She was complaining too much, but millions of women become pregnant don't they?'

(A FATHER)

BECOMING A FATHER

Watching your baby coming into the world is the most incredible experience. The midwives will give you the baby to hold. Some men feel afraid of hurting such a tiny creature. Don't be. Hold the baby close to your body. Feel the softness of the head against your cheek.

Many fathers experience very strong emotions; some cry. It can be very difficult to go home and rest after such an intense experience, so think through what your needs might be at this time. Sleep if you can. You need to recover from the birth too and, when the baby comes home (if the birth took place in hospital), you can expect broken nights for some time to come.

BRINGING THEM HOME

You may find that relatives and friends are able to help in the early days so that your partner can rest and feed your baby. This is especially necessary after a difficult birth. However, you may live far from relatives and she may only have you. It's a good idea to have a week or so off work if you can. Think about the following:

- too many visitors may exhaust her;

- you could look after the baby so she can get a good rest each day;

- take over the basic housework, but don't feel you must keep the place spotless. No one should expect it;

- try to use this time to get to know your baby. You could learn to change nappies and bath your baby as well as cuddling and

playing with him or her. If your partner is breastfeeding you could bring her a snack and a drink while she feeds the baby. If bottle feeding, you could sterilise and make up the bottles (see page 70) and share the feeding;

- when you go back to work you may have to make up for her lost earnings, but keep overtime to a minimum. You will want to continue learning about your baby and being there so you can watch your child grow and develop;

- be considerate about sex. It may take many weeks to months before she stops feeling sore. You could discuss other ways of showing your love for each other until intercourse is comfortable.

FEELING LOW

Some mothers become depressed and need a lot of extra support, both practical and emotional (see **Postnatal depression,** page 113). You may also get depressed. Your partner is facing the biggest changes but that doesn't mean that you should ignore your own feelings. You need support too. Keep talking and listening to each other, talk to friends too, and be patient – life will get easier in time.

7 Antenatal care and antenatal classes

Throughout your pregnancy you will have regular care, either at a hospital antenatal clinic or with your own GP or community midwife. This is to check that you and the baby are well and so that any problems can be picked up as early as possible. This is the time to get answers to any questions or worries and to discuss plans for your baby's birth.

THE FIRST VISIT

Most women have their first, and longest, antenatal check-up around the 8th to 12th week of pregnancy. The earlier you go the better. You should allow plenty of time as you will probably see a midwife and a doctor, and may be offered an ultrasound scan

QUESTIONS

You can expect a lot of questions on your health, on any illnesses and operations you have had, and on any previous pregnancies or miscarriages. You will be asked for any information you have on your own family and your partner's family (whether there are twins on your side or any inherited illness, for example). You will also be asked about your ethnic origin. This is because certain inherited conditions that need attention in early pregnancy are more common in some ethnic groups.

There may also be questions about your work or your partner's work and what kind of accommodation you live in, to see if there is anything about your circumstances that might affect your pregnancy.

All this information will help to build up a picture of you and your pregnancy so that any special risks can be spotted and support provided.

The midwife or doctor will want to know the date of the first day of your last period, to work out when the baby is due. You will probably want to ask a lot of questions yourself. This is a good opportunity and it often helps if you can write down what you want to say in advance, as it's easy to forget once you are there. It's important to find out what you want to know and to express your own feelings and preferences.

LET YOUR MIDWIFE OR DOCTOR KNOW IF:

- *there were any complications in a previous pregnancy or delivery, such as pre-eclampsia or premature delivery;*

- *you are being treated for a chronic disease such as diabetes or high blood pressure;*

- *you have previously had a baby with an abnormality, for example spina bifida, or there is a family history of an inherited disease such as thalassaemia or cystic fibrosis.*

Remember that, if you're working, you have the right to paid time off for your antenatal care (see page 129).

IF YOU'RE GOING TO HAVE YOUR BABY IN HOSPITAL:

your GP or midwife will write or give you a letter for the hospital. Antenatal care varies around the country. In some areas, the first (booking) appointment is at the hospital then all or most subsequent appointments are with the GP or community midwife unless the pregnancy is complicated, when all appointments are at the hospital. In other areas, all care is given by the GP and/or midwife unless there is a reason for referral to the hospital antenatal clinic.

IF YOU'RE GOING TO HAVE YOUR BABY IN A GP/MIDWIFE UNIT OR AT HOME:

then you will probably go to your own GP and community midwife for most of your antenatal care. You may need to visit the hospital for an initial assessment and perhaps for an ultrasound scan or for special tests. Sometimes your midwife may visit you at home.

WEIGHT

You'll be weighed. From now on, your weight gain will probably be checked regularly, although this is not done everywhere. Most women put on between 10–12.5 kg (22–28 lbs) in pregnancy, most of it after the 20th week. Read pages 8-10 on what to eat in pregnancy, and take regular exercise. Much of the extra weight is due to the baby growing, but your body will also be storing fat ready to make breast milk after the birth.

HEIGHT

Your height will also be measured on the first visit because it is a rough guide to the size of your pelvis. Some small women have small pelvises and will need to discuss their baby's delivery with their doctor or midwife.

GENERAL PHYSICAL EXAMINATION

The doctor will check your heart and lungs and make sure your general health is good.

URINE

You will be asked to give a sample of urine each time you visit. This will be checked for a number of things including:

- **sugar** – pregnant women may have sugar in their urine from time to time but, if it is found repeatedly, you will be checked for diabetes. Some women develop a type of diabetes in pregnancy known as 'gestational diabetes' which can be controlled during pregnancy usually by a change of diet and, possibly, insulin. The condition usually disappears once the baby is born;

- **protein**, or 'albumin' in your urine may show that there is an infection that needs to be treated. It may also be a sign of pregnancy-induced hypertension (see **High blood pressure** on page 80).

BLOOD PRESSURE

Your blood pressure will be taken at every antenatal visit. A rise in blood pressure later in pregnancy could be a sign of pre-eclampsia (see page 80).

TESTS

A number of tests will be offered at your first visit, and some of these will be repeated at later visits. You are under no obligation to have any test, although they are all done to help make your pregnancy safer or to help assess the well being of your baby. Discuss the reasons for tests with your midwife or doctor so that you can make an informed choice about whether or not to have them. Ask to have the results explained to you if you do decide to go ahead.

BLOOD TESTS

You will be offered a blood test which will check:

- **your blood group**;

- **whether your blood is rhesus negative or positive** – a few mothers are rhesus negative. Usually this is not a worry for the first pregnancy. Some rhesus negative mothers will need an injection after the birth of their first baby to protect their next baby from anaemia. In some units, rhesus negative mothers are given injections called 'anti-D' at 28 and 34 weeks as well as after the birth of their baby. This is quite safe and is done to make sure that the blood of future babies is not affected by rhesus disease;

- **whether you are anaemic** – if you are, you will probably be given iron and folic acid tablets to take. Anaemia makes you tired and less able to cope with losing blood at delivery.

- **your immunity to rubella** (German measles) – if you get rubella in early pregnancy, it can seriously damage your unborn baby. If you are not immune to rubella and come into contact with it, blood tests will show whether you have been infected. If so, you'll be offered the option of ending your pregnancy after discussing the possible problems your baby might have;

- **for syphilis** – it is vital to detect and treat any woman who has this sexually transmitted infection as early as possible;

- **for hepatitis B** – this is a virus which causes liver disease and may infect the baby if you are a carrier of the virus or are infected during pregnancy. The baby can be immunised at birth to prevent infection.

HIV BLOOD TEST

HIV is the virus that causes AIDS. You won't be tested routinely for HIV infection, but some hospitals are carrying out unlinked anonymous surveys to try to find out just how widespread HIV is in the population. If your hospital is one of these, then leaflets and posters explaining the survey should be on display.

Anonymous testing involves testing some of the blood from the routine checks described above, for HIV antibodies. All specimens have any details which could identify the woman permanently removed before testing so that there is no possibility that your result can be traced back to you. You can ask for your specimen to be excluded from the survey if you wish. You can be sure that the survey will not affect your antenatal care in any way.

In some hospitals (usually those in inner city areas) the prevalence of HIV has been found to be higher than that of the general population through this anonymous testing. A named confidential HIV test is being offered to all women in some of these units, so that interventions known to decrease the risk of the baby being infected can be offered to infected women (see box).

If you think that you may have been at risk of getting HIV, ask your doctor or midwife for the opportunity to discuss HIV testing and counselling. If you're HIV positive, you can talk to someone at Positively Women, an organisation concerned with women and HIV and AIDS (see page 136).

SICKLE CELL DISEASE AND THALASSAEMIA

Sickle cell disease is a blood condition that mainly affects people of African and West Indian origin and, less often, people from India, the Middle East and Mediterranean. Thalassaemia, another blood condition, mainly affects people of Mediterranean and Asian origin. If you, your partner, or your parents originally come from these parts of the world, you'll probably be offered a blood test to find out whether you are a carrier. It is possible for either you or your partner to be a carrier

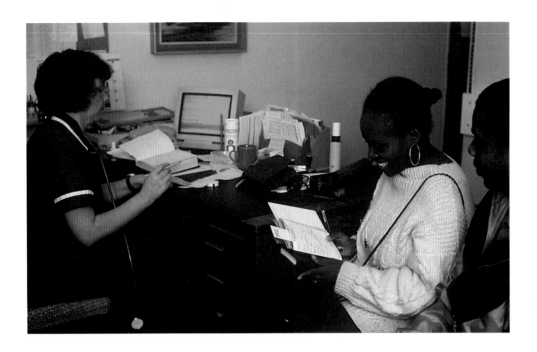

without it affecting your baby at all. But if both of you are carriers, or if either of you suffer from the disease yourself, you should discuss the implications for the baby with your doctor or midwife. Or contact the Sickle Cell Society or the UK Thalassaemia Society (see page 136).

INTERNAL EXAMINATION

Occasionally, the doctor might consider it necessary to do an internal examination. Discuss the reasons for this with the doctor. By putting one or two fingers inside your vagina and pressing the other hand on your abdomen, your doctor can judge the age of your baby. Most doctors prefer to use an ultrasound scan for this purpose (see page 52) either at the first or a later visit.

CERVICAL SMEAR

You will be offered a cervical smear test now if you haven't had one in the last three years. The test detects early changes in the cervix (the neck of the womb) which could later lead to cancer if left untreated. By sliding an instrument called a speculum into your vagina, the doctor can look at your cervix. A smear is then taken from the surface of the cervix and will be examined under a microscope. The test may feel a bit uncomfortable but it is not painful and won't harm the growing baby.

HERPES

If you, or your partner, have ever had genital herpes, or you get your first attack of genital blisters or ulcers during your pregnancy, let your doctor or midwife know. This is important because herpes can be dangerous for your newborn baby and he or she may need special monitoring and possibly treatment.

LATER VISITS

Later visits are usually shorter. Your urine and blood pressure, and often your weight, will be checked. Your abdomen will be felt to check the baby's position and growth. And the doctor or midwife will listen to your baby's heartbeat. You can also ask questions or talk about anything that is worrying you. Talking is as much a part of antenatal care as all the tests and examinations.

From now on, antenatal checks will usually be every four weeks until 28 weeks, every two weeks until 36 weeks, and then every week until the baby is born. If your pregnancy is uncomplicated, you may be offered the option of less frequent antenatal appointments. If you can't keep an antenatal appointment, let the clinic, GP or midwife know, and make another appointment.

ULTRASOUND SCAN

This test uses sound waves to build up a picture of the baby in the womb. Most hospitals will offer women at least one ultrasound scan during their pregnancy. An ultrasound scan can be used to:

- check the baby's measurements – this gives a better idea of the baby's age and can help decide when your baby is likely to be born. This can be useful if you are unsure about the date of your last period;

- check whether you are carrying more than one baby;

- detect some abnormalities, particularly in the baby's head or spine;

- show the position of the baby and the placenta. In some cases, for example where the placenta is low in late pregnancy, special care may be needed at delivery or a Caesarean section may be advised;

- check that the baby is growing and developing normally.

The scan is completely painless, has no known serious side effects on mothers or their babies (although research is continuing), and can be carried out at any stage of pregnancy. Most hospitals scan all women at 18 to 20 weeks to check for certain abnormalities.

You will probably be asked to drink a lot of fluid before you have the scan. A full bladder pushes your womb up and this gives a better picture. You then lie on your back and some jelly is put on your abdomen. An instrument is passed backwards and forwards over your skin and high frequency sound is beamed through your abdomen into the womb. The sound is reflected back and creates a picture which is shown on a TV screen. It can be very exciting to see a picture of your own baby before birth, often moving about inside.

Ask for the picture to be explained to you if you can't make it out. It may be possible for your partner to come with you and see the scan. Many couples feel that this helps to make the baby real for them both. Ask if it's possible to have a copy of the picture. (There may be a small charge for this.)

If you feel doubtful about having a scan, talk it over with your GP, midwife or obstetrician.

TESTS TO DETECT ABNORMALITIES IN THE BABY

It is important to realise that no test can guarantee that your baby will be born without abnormality. No test is 100% accurate and some abnormalities may remain undetected. When you are deciding whether or not to have a test, think what you might do if the test suggests that your baby has an abnormality. Since amniocentesis and chorion villus sampling (CVS) carry a risk of miscarriage, you may decide not to have these tests if you would choose to continue with the pregnancy. Having a test, however, may reassure you that your baby is likely to be born healthy, allow you to consider the termination of an affected baby or give you time to prepare for the arrival of a baby with special needs. Discuss the issues with your partner, midwife, doctor and friends.

The tests below are designed to detect **structural abnormalities** like spina bifida or **genetic disorders** like Down's syndrome. Chromosomes are the structures within every cell of a person's body which carry the individual genetic code or recipe to make that person. Down's syndrome is caused by an abnormal number of chromosomes. Conditions like cystic fibrosis and achondroplasia (dwarfism) are caused by abnormalities within the chromosomes (so causing a 'mistake' in the recipe). Talk to your midwife, GP or obstetrician about the following tests as they are not available in all hospitals.

ULTRASOUND (see also page 52)

Since ultrasound provides an image of the baby in the womb, it detects **structural abnormalities**, particularly of the spine and head. Recently, however, it has been found to be useful in screening for Down's syndrome and some other abnormalities of chromosome number. Several research studies have shown that the thickness of the 'nuchal fold' at the back of the baby's neck is related to the risk of Down's syndrome. An ultrasound scan at 10 to 13 weeks enables a measurement to be taken. This measurement then allows a risk factor to be calculated. The **nuchal translucency scan** is not widely available because its reliability requires further evaluation.

ALPHA-FETOPROTEIN (AFP) TEST

This test is performed at about 15 to 20 weeks to find out the level of alpha-fetoprotein (AFP) in your blood. This protein is made by your baby and passes into your blood during pregnancy. High levels are associated with spina bifida and so an ultrasound scan will then be offered to check for this. High levels may be seen in normal pregnancy and also in twin pregnancy. Low levels of AFP are associated with Down's syndrome pregnancies. Ultrasound and amniocentesis will then be suggested to achieve a diagnosis.

Some hospitals routinely offer the AFP test to all women; others don't, or restrict the test to older women since the risk of Down's syndrome, and some other abnormalities of chromosome number, increases with age.

(see page 134)

IF A TEST DETECTS AN ABNORMALITY:

you may like to contact the appropriate organisation (see page 134) for further information. They may be able to put you in touch with parents who have decided to continue with a pregnancy in which an abnormality has been detected. **SATFA** *(Support Around Termination For Abnormality) will offer support and information if you are considering termination for abnormality.*

SERUM SCREENING

This is the term used for a blood test which screens for Down's syndrome. It combines the AFP result (and so gives information about the risk of spina bifida) with the measurement of other blood chemicals to give the relative risk of having a baby with Down's syndrome. There are various tests available ('double test', 'triple plus test' etc.) which differ slightly from each other, but they are all types of serum screening.

Some units give the result as 'screen negative' or 'screen positive'. A negative result means that Down's syndrome is unlikely. A positive result means that Down's syndrome is more likely. An amniocentesis will be suggested to give more information. Other units give a numerical result, for example 1:250 risk of Down's syndrome. You may like to compare this risk to that for your age (about 1:900 at 30) or to the risk of miscarriage with amniocentesis (about 1:100). Your doctor or midwife will explain the significance of the result to you. If the test is not available locally on the NHS, you may be able to obtain a test privately.

AMNIOCENTESIS

This test may be offered from 14 weeks of pregnancy:

- to women who have an AFP or serum screening result which indicates an increased risk of Down's syndrome;

- when an ultrasound scan detects an abnormality which is associated with a genetic disorder;

- when a woman's past or family history suggests that there may be a risk of her baby having a genetic disorder such as Down's syndrome;

- occasionally when a high AFP suggests that the baby has spina bifida. Ultrasound is more commonly used to make this diagnosis.

An ultrasound scan is performed to check the position of the baby and placenta. Whilst continuing to scan with the ultrasound probe, a fine needle is passed through the wall of the abdomen into the amniotic fluid which surrounds the baby. A small sample of this fluid is drawn off and sent to the laboratory for testing. Most women feel only mild discomfort.

Within the fluid are cells which contain the same chromosomes as the baby. Looking at these chromosomes is a complex process which is why the results take up to three weeks. This test will reveal your baby's sex. Tell your doctor whether or not you want to know what it is. Some disorders such as haemophilia and muscular dystrophy are only found in boys (although girls may carry the disorder in their chromosomes and pass it on to their sons). Tell your doctor if these or other genetic disorders run in your family as it may then be important to know your baby's sex.

Amniocentesis is associated with a 1% risk of miscarriage. That is, one test in a hundred will result in pregnancy loss. When deciding whether or not to go ahead with this test try to balance the risk of miscarriage against the value of the result to you. Remember that a normal result only reassures you about the number of chromosomes unless specific tests for disorders such as cystic fibrosis have been done. The result for spina bifida (level of AFP in the amniotic fluid) only takes a few days.

CHORION VILLUS SAMPLING (CVS)

This test is usually only available in large hospitals but smaller units are able to refer to these units if necessary. It tests for genetic disorders. It does not give information about spina bifida.

CVS can be carried out earlier than amniocentesis at around ten weeks but carries a higher risk of miscarriage, at about 2–3%. CVS before ten weeks has been associated

with a slightly increased risk of limb deformities. Women at risk of having a child with an inherited disorder such as cystic fibrosis or muscular dystrophy may accept the increased risk of miscarriage in order to obtain an earlier diagnosis.

The test takes 10 to 20 minutes and may be a little uncomfortable. Using ultrasound as a guide, a fine needle is passed through the woman's abdomen, or sometimes a fine tube through the vagina and cervix, into the womb. A tiny piece of the developing placenta, known as chorionic tissue, is withdrawn. Again, the chromosomes in the cells of this tissue are looked at. The results take up to two weeks.

If you feel the test would be helpful, talk over the matter carefully with your GP or midwife early in your pregnancy or before conception, as well as with your partner or a close friend. You can also contact your regional genetic centre direct (telephone the Genetic Interest Group for details of your nearest centre, see page 135).

MAKING THE MOST OF ANTENATAL CARE

'There were some things that really annoyed me – the gowns, and the lavatories, and one midwife who called everyone "sweetie". But there were other things I wouldn't have missed – like hearing my baby's heart beating, and well, just knowing she was alright. Knowing I was alright too, come to that.'

'I think it's up to you to make the most of it. You can find out a lot, but you have to ask. When your blood pressure's taken, you have to say, "Is that alright?". Then they'll tell you. And if it's not alright, you have to ask why not, and talk about it. It's the same for everything. It's not being a nuisance, it's being interested. I think the staff like it if you're interested.'

Having regular antenatal care is important for your health and the health of your baby. However, sometimes antenatal visits can seem quite an effort. If the clinic is busy or short-staffed you may have to wait a long time and, if you have small children with you, this can be very exhausting. By increasing the number of women that are cared for by their GP and community midwife, antenatal care should become more convenient. Try to plan ahead to make your visits easier and come prepared to wait. Here are some suggestions.

- In some clinics you can buy refreshments. If not, take a snack with you if you are likely to get hungry.

- Write a list of any questions you want to ask and take it with you to remind you. Make sure you get answers to your questions or the opportunity to discuss any worries. Sometimes this can take quite a lot of determination.

- If your partner is free he may be able to go with you. He'll be able to support you in discussing any worries or in finding out what you want to know. It will also help him to feel more involved in your pregnancy.

- If you regularly wait for long periods at your clinic, bring this to the attention of the hospital management. They have a responsibility to ensure that Patient's Charter standards are met.

YOUR ANTENATAL NOTES

At your first antenatal visit, your doctor or midwife will enter your details in a record book and add to them at each visit. Many hospitals ask women to look after these notes themselves. Other hospitals keep the notes and give you a card which records your details. Take your notes or card with you wherever you go. Then, if you need medical attention while you are away from home, you will have the information that's needed with you.

The page opposite gives a sample of the information your card or notes may contain, as each clinic has its own system. Always ask your doctor or midwife about anything on your card which you would like to have explained.

R.O.L. or R.O.T.   L.O.P

L.O.A.

L.O.L.
or
L.O.T   R.O.A.   R.O.P.

POSITION

The above abbreviations are used to describe the way the baby is lying – facing sideways, for example, or frontwards or backwards. Ask your midwife to explain the way your baby is lying.

RELATION TO BRIM
At the end of pregnancy your baby's head (or bottom, or feet if it is in the breech position) will start to move into your pelvis. Doctors and midwives 'divide' the baby's head into 'fifths' and describe how far it has moved down into the pelvis by judging how many 'fifths' of the head they can feel above the brim (the bone at the front). They may say that the head is 'engaged' this is when $2/5$ or less of the baby's head can be felt above the brim. This may not happen until you are in labour. If all of the baby's head can be felt above the brim, this is described as 'free' or $5/5$.

OEDEMA
This is another word for swelling, most often of the feet and hands. Usually it is nothing to worry about, but tell your doctor or midwife if it suddenly gets worse as this may be a sign of pre-eclampsia (see page 80).

BLOOD PRESSURE
(BP) This usually stays at about the same level throughout pregnancy. If it goes up a lot in the last half of pregnancy, it may be a sign of pre-eclampsia which can be dangerous for you and your baby (see page 80).

FETAL HEART
'FHH' or just 'H' means 'fetal heart heard'. 'FMF' means 'fetal movement felt'.

Hb
This stands for 'haemoglobin'. It is tested in your blood sample to check you are not anaemic.

DATE	WEEKS	WEIGHT	URINE ALB SUGAR	BP	HEIGHT FUNDUS	PRESENTATION AND POSITION	RELATION OF PP TO BRIM	FH	OEDEMA	Hb	NEXT	SIG.	NOTES
15/6/97	13	58kg	nil	110/60	15	-	-	-		12.0	20/7	CS	u/s arranged for 17/7 to check maturity
20/7/97	18	59.2	Nil	125/60	18-20	-	-	FMF	-	-	21/8	CS	
21/8/97	22	61Kg	Nil	135/65	20	22	-	-	-	-	18/9	CS	taking iron
18/9/97	26	64Kg	Nil	125/75	24-26	ceph	-	H	-	11.2	28/10	CS	
28/10/97	30	66Kg	Nil	125/70	30	ceph	5/5	FHH	-	-	27/11	CS	Mat B1 given, Hb taken
27/11/97	34	-	Nil	115/75	34	ceph	4/5	FHH	-	11.0	15/12	CS	

DATE
This is the date of your antenatal visit.

WEEKS
This refers to the length of your pregnancy in weeks from the date of your last menstrual period.

PRESENTATION
This refers to which way up the baby is. Up to about 30 weeks, the baby moves about a lot. Then it usually settles into its head downward position, ready to be born head first. This is recorded as 'Vx' (vertex) or 'C' or 'ceph' (cephalic). Both words mean the top of the head. If your baby stays with its bottom downwards, this is a breech ('Br') presentation. 'PP' means presenting part, that is the bit of the baby that is coming first. 'Tr' (transverse) means your baby is lying across your tummy.

URINE
These are the results of your urine tests for protein and sugar. '+' or 'Tr' means a quantity (or trace) has been found. 'Alb' stands for 'albumin', a name for one of the proteins detected in urine. 'Nil' or a tick or 'NAD' all mean the same: nothing abnormal discovered. 'Ketones' may be found if you have not eaten recently or have been vomiting.

HEIGHT OF FUNDUS
By gently pressing on your abdomen, the doctor or midwife can feel your womb. Early in pregnancy the top of the womb, or 'fundus', can be felt low down, below your navel. Towards the end it is well up above your navel, just under your breasts. So the height of the fundus is a guide to how many weeks pregnant you are.
This column gives the length of your pregnancy, in weeks, estimated according to the position of the fundus. The figure should be roughly the same as the figure in the 'weeks' column. If there's a big difference (say, more than two weeks), ask your doctor about it. Sometimes the height of the fundus may be measured with a tape measure and the result entered on your card in centimetres.

WHO'S WHO

Many mothers would like to be able to get to know the people who care for them during pregnancy and the birth of their baby. The NHS is now working to achieve this. However, you may still find that you see a number of different carers. Professionals should, of course, introduce themselves and explain what they do but, if they forget, don't hesitate to ask. It may help to make a note of who you have seen and what they have said in case you need to discuss any point later on. These are the people you're most likely to meet. Some may have students with them who are being trained and you will be asked if you mind them being present.

- **A midwife** is specially trained to care for mothers and babies throughout normal pregnancy, labour and after the birth, and therefore provides all care for the majority of women at home or in hospital. Increasingly, midwives will be working both in hospital and in the community so that they can provide better continuity of care. You should know the name of the midwife who is res-ponsible for your midwifery care.

- **A hospital midwife or doctor** will probably see you each time you go to a hospital antenatal clinic. A midwife will look after you during labour and will probably deliver your baby, if your delivery is normal. If any complications develop during your pregnancy or delivery, a doctor will become more closely involved with your care. You and your baby will be cared for by midwives on the postnatal ward until you go home. You will probably also meet student midwives and student doctors.

- **A community midwife** will probably get to know you before your baby is born and will visit you at home, after you leave hospital during the early weeks. Community midwives are sometimes attached to GPs' practices and may be involved in giving antenatal care. They are also involved in delivering babies in community and GP/midwife units and are responsible for home deliveries. Some community midwives also accompany women into the hospital maternity unit to be with them for the birth.

- **Your general practitioner (GP)** can help you to plan your antenatal care. This may be given at the hospital, but it is quite often shared with the GP. Sometimes the GP may be responsible for all your antenatal care. If you have your baby in a GP/midwife unit or at home, your GP may be involved in your baby's birth. If your baby is born in hospital, your GP will be notified of your baby's birth and will arrange to see you soon after you return home. Don't forget to register your baby with your GP.

- **An obstetrician** is a doctor specialising in the care of women during pregnancy, labour and soon after the birth. If you are having a hospital birth you will be under the care of a consultant and the doctors on his or her own team, together with other professionals such as midwives. In some hospitals you will routinely see an obstetrician; in others, your midwife or GP will refer you for an appointment if they have a particular concern such as previous complications of pregnancy or labour or chronic illness. If everything is straightforward, a midwife will usually deliver your baby. You should ask to see your consultant if you wish to discuss any matter you think is important.

● **A paediatrician** is a doctor specialising in the care of babies and children. The paediatrician may check your baby after the birth to make sure all is well and will be present when your baby is born if you have had a difficult labour. If your baby should have any problems, you will be able to talk this over with the paediatrician. If your baby is born at home or your stay in hospital is short, you may not see a paediatrician at all. Your GP can check that all is well with you and your baby.

● **An obstetric physiotherapist** is specially trained to help you cope with the physical changes of pregnancy, childbirth and afterwards. Some attend antenatal classes and teach antenatal exercises, relaxation and breathing, active positions and other ways you can help yourself during pregnancy and labour. Afterwards, they advise on postnatal exercises to tone up your muscles again. When no obstetric physiotherapist is available your midwife can help you with these exercises.

● **Health visitors** are specially trained nurses concerned with the health of the whole family. You may meet yours before the birth of your baby. The health visitor will contact you to arrange a home visit when your baby is ten days old to offer help and support. You may continue to see your health visitor either at home, or at your Child Health Clinic, health centre or GP's surgery, depending on where they are based.

ANTENATAL CLASSES

Think about what you hope to gain from antenatal classes so that, if there is a choice, you can find the sort of class that suits you best. You need to start making enquiries early in pregnancy so that you can be sure of getting a place in the class you choose. You can go to more than one class. Ask your midwife, or health visitor, your GP, or the local branch of the National Childbirth Trust (see page 134).

'My midwife told me about a class specially for teenagers. It was great being with girls my age.'

'It really helped me to make up my mind about how I wanted to have my baby.'

Antenatal classes can help to prepare you for your baby's birth and for looking after and feeding your baby. They can also help you to keep yourself fit and well during pregnancy. They are often called parentcraft classes and may cover relaxation and breathing, and antenatal exercise. They're a good chance to meet other parents, to talk about things that might be worrying you and to ask questions – and to make new friends. They are usually informal and fun.

You may be able to go to some introductory classes on babycare early in pregnancy. Otherwise, many classes will start about eight to ten weeks before your baby is due. Classes are normally held once a week, either during the day or in the evening and last one or two hours. Some classes are for expectant women only. Others will welcome partners, either to all the sessions or to some of them, or you can go alone or with a friend. In some areas there are classes especially for women whose first language is not English, classes for single mothers and classes for teenagers. The kinds of topics covered by antenatal classes are:

- health in pregnancy

- what happens during labour and birth

- coping with labour and information about pain relief

- exercises to keep you fit during pregnancy and help you in labour

- relaxation

- caring for your baby, including feeding

Now, relax...

- your own health after the birth

- 'refresher classes' for those who have already had a baby

- emotions surrounding pregnancy, birth and the early postnatal period.

Some classes will try to cover all these topics. Others will concentrate more on certain aspects, such as exercises and relaxation or babycare.

The number of different antenatal classes available varies very much from place to place. Classes may be run by your hospital, by your local midwives or health visitors, by your own GP or health centre. The National Childbirth Trust also runs classes, usually in the evenings and in the leader's home. The groups tend to be smaller and may go into more depth.

Antenatal classes may give you the opportunity to get to know some of the professionals involved in your care and to ask questions and talk over any worries you may have. You can find out about arrangements for labour and birth and the sort of choices available to you. This can help you in thinking about making your own birth plan (see page 35). You'll usually be able to look round the labour and postnatal wards. You may also be able to meet some of the people who will be looking after you when the time comes for your baby to be born.

Classes can give you confidence as well as information. You'll be able to talk over any worries and discuss your plans, not just with professionals, but with other parents as well.

Speak to your community midwife if you can't go to classes. The midwife may have videos to lend you or you may be able to hire or buy one.

'It was great meeting people who were going through the same things I was.'

'It was brilliant having classes in the evening because it meant Phil could help me during labour.'

'Being shown the delivery suite helped us – just knowing what to expect made it less scary.'

Classes may be available in your area for specific groups such as single women and teenagers. Ask your midwife for details.

8 The feeding question

'It was so easy. I suppose it took me about a couple of weeks to get used to it, and from then on I just didn't have to think. It was the one thing that wasn't any effort at all.'

'Breastfeeding was so difficult what with one thing and another – first the baby was ill, then me. I'd be crying. The baby would be crying and hungry. So we started on the bottle and somehow from then on it was alright and I felt much better about it all.'

I t's never too early to start thinking about how you're going to feed your baby. Once your baby is born there will be lots to occupy you! You'll need to discuss it with other people, the baby's father, your midwife, health visitor or other mothers.

Breastfeeding is best for the health of your baby, but it's also important that you feel happy and comfortable about the choice you have made. You can't know in advance what breastfeeding will be like but, knowing that it's best for your baby, you can always decide to breastfeed at first and then change to bottle feeding if it really doesn't work out. It's difficult to change from bottle to breastfeeding. If you don't breastfeed at all you may later regret that you never had the experience.

If you're HIV positive you will be advised not to breastfeed because of the risk of passing the virus on to your baby through the milk. It is a good idea to discuss this with your midwife or doctor.

WATER

You may be advised to give your baby water between feeds if he or she cries, in case the baby is thirsty rather than hungry. This is not necessary. Even in very hot countries no extra water is needed. This is true for both breast and bottle-fed babies. Offer your baby a feed even if she or he has been fed recently. It is important to feed on demand since babies often don't conform to routine. This is particularly important for breastfed babies because they increase the milk supply by increasing the frequency of feeds. If your baby still won't settle, go through the checklist on page 115.

BREASTFEEDING

WHY BREAST IS BEST FOR BABIES

● Breast milk is the only food naturally designed for your baby. It contains the nutrients your baby needs in the right amounts and they are in a form that is very easily absorbed.

● Breast milk contains antibodies and other protective factors which are transferred from you to your baby to help him or her fight against infections. It also helps to build up long-term resistance to infections.

● Breast milk is easily digested and absorbed and is less likely to cause stomach upsets or diarrhoea. It will also help to avoid constipation in your baby.

● Breastfed babies are less likely to get allergies like eczema, for example.

● Breast milk contains growth factors and hormones to assist your baby's development.

WHY BREAST IS BEST FOR MOTHERS

As one mother said, 'It was feeling close, and being together, that was what I liked', but there are other benefits too.

● Breastfeeding costs nothing.

● There's no need to prepare feeds or wash and sterilise bottles.

● Your baby isn't kept waiting for a feed.

● Breastfeeding helps your womb return to its normal size more quickly and, because it uses up calories, it will help you to lose some of the weight gained in pregnancy.

● It's so much easier and more practical in the middle of the night.

'I didn't want to breastfeed. It was as simple as that. The whole idea of it put me off and I just couldn't have done it.'

'I had quite a few problems at first with sore nipples and one thing and another. It made it difficult. I think I'd have given up if it hadn't been for the midwife. She was ever so good. And after a while it all sorted out and now I'm glad I did it.'

NURSING BRAS

A nursing bra will give you support so that you feel more comfortable. Choose adjustable bras because the size of your breasts will change (see page 84). Some women feel more comfortable wearing a nursing bra at night as well.

63

SOME OF YOUR QUESTIONS ANSWERED

Can all women breastfeed?
Almost every woman can breastfeed, but it can sometimes take a little while to get it right. Be patient and ask your midwife or health visitor for help if you need it.

Does breast size matter?
No. All shapes and sizes make milk.

Can flat or inverted nipples be a problem?
Most women with flat or inverted nipples should be able to breastfeed. However, you may need a little extra help in learning to position your baby (see page 66).

Do I need to prepare my breasts for breastfeeding?
Your breasts will prepare themselves naturally, although it's a good idea to try to keep your skin soft and supple, so avoid soaps and sprays that have a drying effect.

If my baby is born prematurely, will it have the energy to suck at the breast?
Maybe not at first, but small babies will benefit if they get some mother's milk as it is exactly right for them. Your milk can be given by bottle, tube or cup, if your baby can't take it directly from your breast.

How can I make sure my partner feels involved?
Breastfeeding is only one way to be close to a baby. Your partner can cuddle and bathe the baby and perhaps give bottles of expressed milk later on.

Can I go out without the baby?
Yes, sometimes. You can express some of your milk and leave it for someone else to give your baby (see page 68).

'I didn't realise that bottle feeding would be so much trouble. It was really hard to find time to sterilise and make up the bottles. My new baby took up all my time.'

'I really enjoy the closeness of breastfeeding and my partner says it makes him feel so proud, watching us together.'

Is it worth breastfeeding if I am going back to work soon?
Yes. The early weeks, while you are at home, are the time when breast milk does the most good. After that you can express your breast milk or use powdered milk for your baby while you are at work and continue to breastfeed at other times.

What about feeding my baby in front of friends or in public?
You may be quite happy about feeding in front of others. If you feel uneasy, you could feed the baby discreetly under a loose top, T-shirt or half-unbuttoned blouse. Don't be embarrassed to ask if there's a mother and baby room when you're out.

Breastfeeding a baby can be a great pleasure. Even if it doesn't go well for you at the start, it's still worth working at. Although problems with breastfeeding, even fairly small problems, can be quite upsetting, they can almost always be overcome.

You can get help from:

- your midwife or health visitor

- a breastfeeding counsellor or support group. Contact your local branch of the National Childbirth Trust, or the La Leche League (page 134). These organisations give help and support through other mothers who have experience of breastfeeding.

Don't worry if other mothers seem to be doing things differently. It is important to have confidence in yourself and your baby so that together you can work out what is best for both of you.

THE FIRST FEW DAYS

In the beginning, it can seem that you are doing nothing but feeding, but gradually your baby will settle into a pattern of feeding. Try to relax into it and take each day as it comes.

For the first few days after birth your breasts produce a special food called **colostrum**, which looks like rich creamy milk and is sometimes quite yellow in colour. This contains all the food your baby needs, as well as antibodies which pass your own resistance to certain infections on to your baby.

After about three days your breasts will begin to produce milk which will look quite thin compared with colostrum. The milk now varies according to the needs of your baby. The **fore milk**, which your baby takes first, is thirst quenching and means your baby gets a drink at the start of every feed. A breastfed baby doesn't need any other drinks (including infant teas or juices), even in hot weather, as long as you feed whenever the baby asks. The fore milk is then followed by the richer **hind milk**. This is the food part of the feed and contains the calories your baby needs. This is why you shouldn't restrict the length of feeds. Your breasts may become very large and heavy for a while and may feel uncomfortable, or even painful, at first.

Milk may leak from your nipples and you may feel more comfortable wearing breast pads. Change them frequently. Avoid plastic backs. Or you can use clean cotton hankies, and at night you could put a clean towel under you instead of wearing pads.

Gradually the amount of milk you produce will settle down and your breasts will begin to feel normal again. If you are very uncomfortable, ask your midwife for help.

HOW BREASTFEEDING WORKS

Your milk supply
Your breasts produce milk in response to your baby feeding at your breast. The more your baby feeds, the more your body makes milk, provided that your baby is correctly positioned. If you reduce feeding, you will make less milk.

The 'let-down' reflex
Your baby's sucking causes milk to gather behind the nipple, ready for feeding. This is called the 'let-down' reflex; some mothers feel it as a tingling sensation. You will see quick sucks change to deep swallows once the milk has begun to flow. Babies pause while they wait for more milk to be 'delivered'.

If you're breastfeeding and you're on Income Support or Income-based Jobseeker's Allowance you can get tokens for free milk for yourself and vitamins for you and your baby (see page 128) which may be recommended from six months or earlier in some cases.

'I wasn't sure if I'd be able to breastfeed. My mum bottle fed me so she couldn't help. Once I got going though, it was so easy. I can't think now why I was so unsure at first.'

IMPORTANT POINTS TO REMEMBER

- *If your baby just feeds on the nipple, he or she will get very little milk and you may become sore.*

- *If feeding feels wrong or hurts or your baby doesn't seem to be feeding properly, stop the feed. Break the suction by putting your little finger into the corner of your baby's mouth. Adjust the position and start again.*

- *Breastfeeding may be a little uncomfortable at first, but this will soon ease as you and your baby become accustomed to this new skill.*

HOW TO BREASTFEED

This is a new skill, so you should ask your midwife to show you how. The following hints will give you a few basic ideas.

- First find a comfortable position, either sitting upright, well supported or lying down.

- Then turn your baby towards you with the head and shoulders opposite your breast and the nose opposite your nipple. Support your baby with a hand across the shoulders not behind the head.

- Now brush your baby's lips against your nipple to get his or her mouth open really wide, then draw your baby to your breast quickly. If you gently stroke down your breast towards the nipple to express a little milk, your baby may find it easier to latch on. If your baby is correctly positioned, there will be more of your areola (the brown skin around the nipple) showing above the top lip than below the bottom lip.

- Start each feed on alternate breasts. Let your baby decide when he or she has finished the first breast before switching to the second. Sometimes babies only need one breast at a feed.

- Many babies will develop a pattern of feeding. You should feed your baby on demand and not let the baby wait for a feed or restrict the length of feeds.

HOW OFTEN AND HOW MUCH

It's best to feed when your baby wants to be fed. This might be very often at first, though feeds will become more spaced out as your baby gets older. Some babies settle into their own pattern quite quickly. Others take longer.

From time to time, your baby will have a growth spurt – usually around 10 days, 6 weeks and 12 weeks. When this happens, your baby needs more milk and you may find that feeds are longer and more frequent. Don't panic and feel you need to offer extra bottles of powdered milk. You'll make more milk in response to your baby's demands, but this may take a day or two, so be patient. The frequency and length of feeds will then settle.

The sucking process releases milk to satisfy your baby and stimulates the production of more. When your baby is full up, he or she will stop feeding. Plenty of wet nappies is a good sign that your baby is getting enough fluid. If you're worried, talk to your midwife, health visitor or breastfeeding counsellor.

HOW TO OVERCOME COMMON DIFFICULTIES

The quicker you sort out any difficulties in breastfeeding, the better for you and your baby. So don't hesitate to ask for help immediately. Many women are surprised to find that most problems are quite easily overcome by a slight change to their baby's position when feeding or by feeding their baby more often.

Feeding restlessly
If your baby is restless at the breast and doesn't seem satisfied by feeds, it may be that he or she is sucking on the nipple alone and so not getting enough milk. Ask for help in making sure your baby feeds in the right position.

Engorged breasts
A few days after the birth, your breasts may become very swollen (engorged) and uncomfortable. The answer is to breastfeed. If feeding is difficult for any reason, ask your midwife for help or make sure you have the telephone number of a breastfeeding counsellor. A good supporting bra will help too, but make sure it isn't too tight.

BREASTFEEDING – WHAT TO EAT AND DRINK

Breastfeeding uses up energy and fluid and you may be hungrier and thirstier than usual. Eat and drink when you feel you need to. It will help to keep you going and keep up your milk supply.

Remember, whatever you eat and drink passes into your breast milk. It's a good idea not to drink too much alcohol. A maximum of one or two units once or twice a week is the best advice whilst breastfeeding. And too much coffee or cola may upset you and your baby. You should always ask your doctor, dentist or pharmacist before taking any medicine or remedy, whether it is prescribed or bought over the counter. If you smoke, some of the nicotine will pass into your baby's bloodstream (see page 11).

*Avoid eating peanuts and foods containing peanut products (e.g. peanut butter, **unrefined** groundnut oil, some snacks, etc.) if you, your baby's father or any previous children have a history of hayfever, asthma, eczema or other allergies. This may reduce the risk of your baby developing a potentially serious allergy to peanuts.*

EXPRESSING MILK

Sometimes you may wish to express your breast milk and leave it in a bottle for someone else to give your baby if, for example, you want to go out for the evening. Your midwife, health visitor or breastfeeding counsellor will show you how to do it. You can do it by hand or use a breast pump. There are different types of breast pump, so ask advice on which to choose. If you use a pump, make sure you sterilise it before and after use.

Store the expressed milk in a sterilised bottle with the top screwed on and in the fridge. Never keep for longer than 24 hours. You can also deep freeze expressed milk, but ask for advice on how to store and defrost it safely first.

*'Knowing that my baby was growing and putting on weight because of milk from **me** made me feel really proud.'*

Sore or cracked nipples

If your nipples are sore when you're feeding, your baby's position will need adjusting. If they are cracked, get advice from your midwife, health visitor or GP as cracked nipples can lead to breast infection. The following suggestions may also help:

- keep your nipples dry and expose them to the air as much as you can – try sleeping topless if it's warm enough, with a towel under you if you're leaking milk;

- change your breast pads frequently (use pads without plastic);

- avoid soap as it dries the skin;

- wear a cotton bra which allows air to circulate;

- try squeezing out a drop or two of your milk at the end of a feed and gently rubbing it into your skin.

If you suddenly get sore and pink nipples after any first soreness has passed, you might have an infection known as thrush. Go and see your GP.

Lumpy tender breasts

These are often caused by blocked milk ducts and there are a number of things you can do to help:

- let your baby feed on the tender breast first or, if he or she doesn't want to feed, try expressing some milk;

- while your baby is feeding, gently stroke the lumpy area with your fingertips, smoothing the milk towards your nipple;

- try leaning over your baby as you feed.

It's important to deal with a blocked duct as soon as possible to make sure that it doesn't lead to mastitis.

Mastitis

If you have mastitis your breasts will feel hot and tender and you may feel as though you have flu. If this occurs, continue to breastfeed but get a midwife or health visitor to check your position. Try the suggestions above for lumpy, tender breasts and get lots of rest. Go to bed if you can. See your GP if there is no improvement within six to eight hours as you may need antibiotics to clear the infection. Your doctor can prescribe one which is safe to take whilst breastfeeding.

WIND

Babies may take in air as they feed – bottle-fed babies more than breastfed babies. After a feed, gentle back rubbing with your baby lying against your shoulder or held a little forward on your lap may bring up some wind that would be uncomfortable otherwise. Don't worry if you don't get any up. It is not essential. It may even be that there is none to come. Sometimes a little milk is brought up at the same time. This is known as **posset** and it's normal.

BOTTLE FEEDING

Bottle feeding may seem like hard work at first until you get into a routine of sterilising bottles and preparing feeds. Once you're organised, you'll be able to relax and really enjoy feeding. Feeding is the best time to hold your baby close in your arms and one advantage of bottle feeding is that fathers can share in this enjoyment.

BABY MILK (INFANT FORMULA)

Baby milk, also called infant formula or artificial milk, usually comes in powder form. It is usually cow's milk that has been specially treated so that babies can digest it. And it has the right balance of vitamins and minerals for a young baby. Baby milks based on soya protein are also available but they are not usually given at this young age.

Ordinary cow's milk, condensed milk, evaporated milk, dried milk, goat's milk, or any other type of milk should never be given to a baby. They are not suitable. If you have any worries about the baby milk you are giving your baby, ask advice from your midwife, health visitor or GP.

There are a number of different brands of baby milk available in the shops. 'Ready-to-feed' baby milks in cartons are also available in some places. This is generally more expensive than powdered milk but may be useful in an emergency or if you're away from home. Once opened, the carton should be stored in the fridge and thrown away after 24 hours.

Although formula milk contains vitamins, you may be advised to give your baby vitamin drops from the age of six months onwards, or earlier in some special cases. You can buy these at the Child Health Clinic.

SOYA-BASED INFANT FORMULAE

If you have chosen to bottle feed but your baby cannot tolerate cow's milk formula, your GP or health visitor may have advised that you feed your baby with a formula based on soya. These formulae are made wholly from plants and so vegan parents may prefer to use them instead of cow's milk formulae. Remember though that breast milk is the best food for your baby.

There has recently been some concern over phytoestrogens, a **natural** component of the soya bean. There is no evidence at present that feeding your baby with soya based formulae will cause any problems, but research is being undertaken to give a better understanding of the effects phytoestrogens have on the body. If you are using soya based formulae because of cow's milk intolerance, remember that babies can grow out of allergies so it may be possible to introduce cow's milk into your baby's diet as he or she gets older. Do not make any changes to your baby's diet without first seeking advice from your GP or health visitor.

'Because Ellen was bottle-fed we both fed her. I used to do it in the evenings and most of the feeds at weekends. We started to do it to give Karen a rest, but in the end I wanted to do it. It brought the baby closer. She's very close to me now.'

(A FATHER)

'When I saw women breastfeeding at my postnatal group, I felt that we'd missed out by using bottles. I'll give breastfeeding a try next time.'

If you are bottle feeding and you're on Income Support or Income-based Jobseeker's Allowance you can get tokens for free milk and vitamins for your baby (see page 128). Vitamins may be recommended from six months or earlier in some cases.

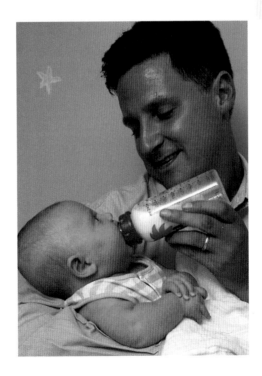

BOTTLES AND TEATS

USING BOTTLED WATER

If you use bottled water to make up a feed, for example on holiday, it must be boiled and then cooled first. Use spring water not mineral water. Use still water, not fizzy.

You'll need at least six bottles and teats. This is to make sure that you always have at least one or two bottles clean, sterilised and ready for use. Ask your midwife, health visitor or other mothers if you want advice on what kind to buy.

You should always buy new teats and it's best if you can buy new bottles too. Check regularly to make sure the bottles are in good condition. If they're badly scratched, you won't be able to sterilise them properly. If in doubt, ask your midwife or health visitor for advice.

MAKING UP THE FEED

When you're preparing formula milk, always **follow the instructions on the tin exactly**. Remember to put the boiled water into the bottle first. The milk powder has been very carefully balanced for your baby, so don't be tempted to add extra powder to make a 'stronger feed' as this could be harmful to your baby. Never use less than instructed and don't add any sugar, honey or anything else.

If you're worried, your midwife or health visitor will advise you how much milk your baby is likely to need. If you make up more than your baby wants, throw away what is left at the end of the feed. You will probably find it suits your routine to make up a number of feeds in advance. Cool the capped bottles quickly under cold running water and put them in the fridge as soon as possible. Don't keep the made up milk for longer than 24 hours.

FEEDING

Your baby will gradually settle into a routine. Babies vary in how often they want to feed and how much they want to take. Some may be content with feeds every three to four hours and others may want smaller quantities more often. Respond to your baby's needs and feed when he or she is hungry, just as you would if you were breastfeeding. In the same way, don't try to force your baby to finish a bottle. He or she may have had enough for the time being or simply want a rest.

The temperature of the milk
Before you start to feed your baby always check that the milk is not too hot by dripping some on the inside of your wrist. Some babies don't mind cold milk. Others prefer it warm. If you want to warm the milk a little, place the bottle upright in some hot water, keeping the teat out of the water. Don't keep the milk warm for more than 20 minutes before the feed as germs can breed in the warmth. Never warm the milk in a microwave oven as this is unsafe. The milk continues to heat for a time after you take it out of the microwave, even though the outside of the bottle may feel cold. The milk inside may be very hot and could scald your baby's mouth.

A comfortable position
Have everything you need ready before you start feeding. Find a comfortable position in which you can hold your baby while you are feeding. Give your baby time. Some babies take some milk, pause for a nap and then wake up for more. So be patient.

The teat

As you feed, keep the bottle tilted so that the teat is always full of milk. Otherwise your baby will be taking in air. If the teat becomes flattened while you are feeding pull gently on the bottle to release the vacuum. If the teat becomes blocked, replace it with another sterile teat. Teats do come in different shapes and with different hole sizes. You may have to try several before you find the one that suits your baby. If the hole is too small your baby will not get enough milk. If it's too big it will come too fast. Check that the teat is not torn or damaged.

After the feed

Gently rub or pat your baby's back for a while to see whether there is any wind to come up. There's no need to overdo this. Wind is not such a problem as many people think. But your baby will probably enjoy the rubbing and closeness to you after the feed.

Don't forget to throw away unused milk in the bottle.

Your midwife or health visitor will chat to you about feeding when they call at your home or you could telephone them or see them at your Child Health Clinic. Talk to them about any worries or problems you may have.

PREPARING A FEED

1 *Make sure your hands are absolutely clean.*

2 *Boil some water in the kettle and let it cool.*

3 *Take a sterilised bottle and teat.*

4 *Take the cooled water and fill the bottle to the right place using the measuring marks.*

5 *Measure the exact amount of powder using the special scoop provided with the milk. Level off the powder in the scoop using a clean dry knife. Don't pack the powder down at all.*

6 *Add the powder to the water in the bottle.*

7 *Screw on the cap and shake well until the powder has dissolved.*

8 *Store the bottle in the fridge if you're not using it straight away.*

CLEANING AND STERILISING

It's important to keep bottles and teats, and other equipment used in feeding, absolutely clean to protect your baby against infection. This means sterilising as well as washing. There are a number of different ways to do this. You can use:

- **a chemical steriliser** – there are several different brands in the shops. They consist of a sterilising tank to which you add cold water and a sterilising tablet or liquid;

- **a steam steriliser** – this is a very quick and efficient method of sterilising;

- **a microwave bottle steriliser** – a microwave alone is not enough to sterilise the bottles without this equipment.

Ask your midwife, health visitor or other mothers about the different methods and which might be most appropriate for you. If you buy equipment, make sure you follow the manufacturer's instructions.

Chemical sterilisation

1 Wash the bottles, teats and other equipment thoroughly in hot water using washing–up liquid. Get rid of every trace of milk using a bottle brush for the inside of the bottles. You may have been advised to use salt to clean the teats, but this is no longer recommended. Squirt water through the teats. This will make sure the holes are clear.

2 Rinse thoroughly in clean running water.

3 To make up the solution, follow the instructions that come with the sterilising tablets or liquid. Put the bottles and teats and other equipment (but nothing metal) in the solution and leave for the time given in the instructions. The tank will have a floating lid that keeps everything under the water or you can use a large plate to keep the bottles immersed. Make sure there are no air bubbles inside the bottles. Put the teats and caps in upside down to prevent air being trapped. Once the equipment is sterilised you should not add new items or the whole solution will be contaminated.

4 Make sure your hands are absolutely clean when you take out the bottles and teats to make up the feeds. When you take out the bottles, shake off the water. It is not necessary to rinse the bottles but if you do, use cooled boiled water. Do not use tap water as this will make them unsterile again.

9 Problems

COMMON MINOR PROBLEMS

Your body has a great deal to do during pregnancy. Sometimes the changes taking place will cause irritation or discomfort, and on occasions they may seem quite alarming. There is rarely any need for alarm but you should mention anything that is worrying you to your doctor or midwife.

If you think that something may be seriously wrong, trust your own judgement and get in touch with your doctor or midwife straight away.

We have listed, in alphabetical order, the changes you are most likely to notice and their causes – where these are known – plus suggestions on how to cope.

BACKACHE

During pregnancy ligaments become softer and stretch to prepare you for labour. This can put a strain on the joints of your lower back and pelvis which can cause backache. As the baby grows, the hollow in your lower back may increase and this may also cause backache.

To avoid backache:

- avoid heavy lifting;

- bend your knees and keep your back straight when lifting or picking something up from the floor;

- if you do have to carry something heavy, hold it close to your body;

- move your feet when turning round to avoid twisting your spine;

- wear flat shoes as these allow your weight to be evenly distributed;

- work at a surface high enough to prevent you stooping;

- try to balance the weight between two baskets if you are carrying shopping;

- sit with your back straight and well supported.

A firm mattress can help to prevent and relieve backache. If your mattress is too soft, a piece of hardboard under the length will make it firmer.

Massage can also help, or you might like to try a support corset – these can be prescribed by the doctor. Make sure you get enough rest, particularly later in pregnancy.

If your backache is very painful, ask your doctor to refer you to an obstetric physiotherapist at your hospital. He or she will be able to give you some advice and suggest some helpful exercises.

CONSTIPATION

You may become constipated very early in pregnancy because of the hormonal changes going on in your body. It will help to:

- make sure you include plenty of fibre in your diet through eating foods like wholemeal breads, wholegrain cereals, fruit and vegetables, and pulses such as beans and lentils;

- exercise regularly to keep your muscles toned up;

- make sure you drink plenty of water;

- avoid iron pills if they cause constipation. Ask your doctor whether you can manage without them or change to a different type. If not, you may have to accept having constipation.

CRAMP

Cramp is a sudden, sharp pain, usually in your calf muscles or feet. It is most common at night, but nobody really knows what causes it. It usually helps if you pull your toes hard up towards your ankle or rub the muscle hard. Regular, gentle exercise in pregnancy, particularly ankle and leg movements, will improve your circulation and may help to prevent cramp occurring.

DISCHARGE FROM BREASTS

You may notice a discharge from your nipples. This is very common and nothing to worry about. However, see your doctor or midwife if it becomes bloodstained.

FAINTNESS

Pregnant women often feel faint. This happens when not enough blood is getting to the brain. If the oxygen level gets too low you may actually faint. It's more common in pregnancy because of hormonal changes taking place in your body. You're most likely to feel faint if you stand still for too long or get up too quickly from a chair or hot bath. It often happens when you are lying on your back.

- Try to get up slowly after sitting or lying down.

- If you feel faint when standing still, find a seat quickly and the faintness will pass. If it doesn't, lie down on your side.

- If you feel faint while lying on your back, turn on to your side. It's better not to lie flat on your back in later pregnancy or during labour.

FEELING HOT IN PREGNANCY

During pregnancy you're likely to feel warmer than normal. This is due to hormonal changes and to an increase in blood supply to the skin. You're also likely to sweat more. It helps if you:

- wear loose clothing made of natural fibres, as these are more absorbent and 'breathe' more than synthetic fibres;

- keep your room cool – consider using an electric fan;

- wash frequently to stay fresh.

HEADACHES

Some pregnant women find they get a lot of headaches. A brisk walk may be all you need, as well as a little more regular rest and relaxation. Although it is wise to avoid drugs in pregnancy, an occasional paracetamol tablet is generally considered safe. If you often have bad headaches, tell your doctor or midwife so that they can advise you. Severe headaches may be a sign of high blood pressure (see page 80).

INDIGESTION AND HEARTBURN

This is partly caused by hormonal changes and later the growing womb pressing on the stomach. If you suffer from indigestion:

- try eating smaller meals more often;

- sit up straight when you are eating as this takes the pressure off your stomach;

- avoid particular foods which cause trouble, for example fried

or highly spiced ones, but make sure you are still eating well (see pages 8-10 for information on healthy eating).

Heartburn is more than just indigestion. It is a strong, burning pain in the chest. It is caused by the valve between your stomach and the tube leading to your stomach relaxing in pregnancy, so that stomach acid passes into the tube. It is often brought on by lying flat. To avoid heartburn you could:

- sleep well propped up – try raising the head of your bed with bricks or have plenty of pillows;

- try drinking a glass of milk – have one by your bed in case you wake with heartburn in the night;

- avoiding eating or drinking for a few hours before you go to bed;

- ask your doctor or midwife for advice;

- don't take antacid tablets or mixture before checking that they are safe in pregnancy.

ITCHING

Mild itching is common in pregnancy because of the increased blood supply to the skin. In late pregnancy the skin of the abdomen is stretched and this may also cause itchiness. Wearing loose clothing may help.

Itching can, however, be a sign of a more serious problem called obstetric cholestasis (see page 80). If itching becomes severe, or you develop a rash or jaundice (yellowing of the whites of the eyes and skin), see your doctor.

Nausea And morning sickness

If you sometimes can't help wetting or soiling yourself, you can get help. Incontinence is a very common problem. It can affect anyone, sometimes during and after pregnancy. In many cases it is curable, so if you've got a problem talk to your doctor, midwife or health visitor, or ring the confidential Continence Foundation Helpline on (0191) 213 0050.

Nausea is very common in the early weeks of pregnancy. Some women feel sick, some are sick. Some feel sick in the mornings, some at other times, some all day long.

The reasons are not fully understood, but hormonal changes in the first three months are probably one cause. Nausea usually disappears around the 12th to 14th week. Nausea can be one of the most trying problems in early pregnancy. It comes at a time when you may be feeling tired and emotional, and when many people around you may not realise you are pregnant and expect you to be your normal self.

- If you feel sick first thing in the morning, give yourself time to get up slowly. If possible, eat something like dry toast or a plain biscuit before you get up. Your partner could bring you some sweet tea.

- Get plenty of rest and sleep whenever you can. Feeling tired can make the sickness worse.

- Eat small amounts often rather than several large meals, but don't stop eating.

- Drink plenty of fluids.

- Ask those close to you for extra support.

- Distract yourself as much as you can. Often the nausea gets worse the more you think about it.

- Avoid the foods and smells that make you feel worse. It helps if someone else can cook but, if not, go for bland, non-greasy foods such as baked potatoes, pasta and milk puddings, which are simple to prepare.

- Wear comfortable clothes. Tight waistbands can make you feel worse.

If you can't keep anything down see your doctor or midwife.

Nose bleeds

Nose bleeds are quite common in pregnancy because of hormonal changes. The nose bleeds are usually short but can be quite heavy. To help the bleeding stop, press the sides of your nose together between your thumb and forefinger just below the bony part of your nose for ten minutes. Repeat for a further ten minutes if this is unsuccessful. As long as you don't lose a lot of blood, there is nothing to worry about. Blow your nose gently and try to avoid explosive sneezes. You may also find that your nose gets more blocked up than usual.

Passing water often

Needing to pass water often is an early sign of pregnancy. Sometimes it continues right through pregnancy. In later pregnancy it's the result of the baby's head pressing on the bladder.

If you find that you're having to get up in the night, you could try cutting out drinks in the late evening but make sure you keep drinking plenty during the day. Later in pregnancy, some women find it helps to rock backwards and forwards while they are on the toilet.

This lessens the pressure of the womb on the bladder so that you can empty it properly. Then you won't need to pass water again quite so soon.

If you have any pain while passing water, or pass any blood, you may have a urine infection which will need treatment. Drink plenty of water to dilute your urine and reduce irritation. You should contact your GP within 24 hours.

Sometimes pregnant women are unable to prevent a sudden spurt of urine or a small leak when they cough, sneeze or laugh, or when moving suddenly or just getting up from a sitting position. This may be temporary because the pelvic floor muscles relax slightly to prepare for the baby's delivery.

The growing baby will increase pressure on the bladder. If you find this a problem, you can improve the situation by doing exercises to tone up your pelvic floor muscles (see page 14). Ask a midwife or obstetric physiotherapist (see page 59) for advice.

PILES

Piles, also known as haemorrhoids, are swollen veins around the back passage which may itch, ache or feel sore. You can usually feel the lumpiness of the piles around the back passage. Piles may also bleed a little and they can make going to the toilet uncomfortable or even painful. They occur in pregnancy because the veins relax under the influence of pregnancy hormones. Piles usually go shortly after delivery. If you suffer from piles you should:

- eat plenty of food that is high in fibre, like wholemeal bread, fruit and vegetables, and you should drink plenty of water. This will prevent constipation, which can make piles worse;

- take regular exercise to improve your circulation;

- avoid standing for long periods;

- sleep with the foot of the bed slightly raised on books or bricks;

- use an ice pack to ease discomfort. Hold this gently against the piles. Or use a cloth wrung out in iced water;

- if the piles stick out, push them gently back inside using a lubricating jelly;

- ask your doctor, midwife or pharmacist if they can suggest a suitable ointment;

- consider giving birth in a position where the pressure on your back passage is reduced – kneeling, for example.

SKIN AND HAIR CHANGES

Hormonal changes taking place in pregnancy will make your nipples and the area around them go darker. Your skin colour may also darken a little, either in patches or all over. Birthmarks, moles and freckles may also darken. Some women develop a dark line running down the middle of their stomachs. These changes will gradually fade after the baby has been born, although your nipples may remain a little darker.

If you sunbathe while you are pregnant, you may find you tan more easily. Protect your skin with a good, high factor sunscreen. Don't stay in the hot sun for very long.

Hair growth is also likely to increase in pregnancy. Your hair may also be greasier. After the baby is born it may seem as if you're losing a lot of hair. In fact, you're simply losing the increase that occurred during pregnancy.

It might be more comfortable to lie on one side with a pillow under your tummy and another between your knees.

SLEEPLESSNESS

Late in pregnancy it can be very difficult to get a good night's sleep. You're uncomfortable lying down, or just when you're beginning to get comfortable you have to get up to go to the toilet. Some women have strange dreams or nightmares about the baby and about the birth. Talking about them can help you. Just because you dream something, it doesn't mean it's going to happen. Relaxation and breathing which are taught in antenatal classes might be helpful.

STRETCH MARKS

These are pink or purplish lines which usually occur on the tummy or sometimes on the upper thighs or breasts. Some women get them, some don't. It depends on your skin type. Some people's skin is more elastic. You are more likely to get stretch marks if your weight gain is more than average.

It's very doubtful whether oils or creams help to prevent stretch marks. After your baby is born the marks should gradually pale and become less noticeable.

SWOLLEN ANKLES, FEET AND FINGERS

Ankles, feet and fingers often swell a little in pregnancy because the body holds more water than usual. Towards the end of the day, especially if the weather is hot or if you have been standing a lot, the extra water tends to gather in the lowest parts of the body. You should:

- try to avoid standing for long periods;

- wear comfortable shoes;

- put your feet up as much as you can – try to rest for an hour a day with your feet higher than your heart;

- try to do your foot exercises (see page 14) – these will help.

TEETH AND GUMS

Bleeding gums are caused by a build-up of plaque (bacteria) on the teeth. During pregnancy, hormonal changes in your body can cause the plaque to make the gums more inflamed. They may become swollen and bleed more easily. To keep your teeth and gums healthy, you should:

- pay special attention to cleaning your teeth. Brush really well to remove all the plaque. Ask your dentist to show you a good brushing method;

- avoid snacking on sugary drinks and foods;

- remember that dental treatment is free while you are pregnant and for a year after your baby's birth, so now is the time for a check-up.

IF YOU AREN'T SLEEPING WELL

- *Try not to let it bother you. Don't worry that it will harm your baby – it won't.*

- *It might be more comfortable to lie on one side with a pillow under your tummy and another between your knees.*

- *Relaxation techniques may help. Your antenatal class (see pages 60-61) may teach relaxation techniques, or you could borrow a cassette from your library.*

- *A warm, milky drink, a warm bath, some gentle exercise or some restful music before bedtime may help.*

- *A rest during the day can help you to feel less tired.*

- *Talk to your partner, a friend, doctor or midwife.*

VAGINAL DISCHARGE

Almost all women have more vaginal discharge in pregnancy. It should be clear and white and it should not smell unpleasant. If the discharge is coloured or smells strange or if you feel itchy or sore, you may have a vaginal infection. Tell your doctor or midwife. The most common infection is thrush which your doctor can treat easily. You can help prevent thrush by wearing loose cotton underwear.

If vaginal discharge, of any colour, increases a lot in later pregnancy, tell your doctor or midwife.

VARICOSE VEINS

Varicose veins are veins which have become swollen. The veins in the legs are most commonly affected. You can also get varicose veins in the vulva (vaginal opening). They usually get better after delivery. You should:

- try to avoid standing for long periods of time;

- try not to sit with your legs crossed;

- try not to put on too much weight as this increases the pressure;

- sit with your legs up as often as you can to ease the discomfort;

- try support tights which may also help support the muscles of your legs – you can buy them at most pharmacists;

- try sleeping with your legs higher than the rest of your body – use pillows under your ankles or put bricks or books under the foot of your bed;

- do foot exercises (see page 14) and other antenatal exercises which will all help your circulation, such as walking, cycling, and swimming.

TIREDNESS

In the early months of pregnancy you may feel tired or even desperately exhausted. The only answer is to try to rest as much as possible. Make time to sit with your feet up during the day and accept any offers of help from colleagues and family. Towards the end of pregnancy, you may feel tired because of the extra weight you are carrying. Make sure you get plenty of rest.

MORE SERIOUS PROBLEMS

SLOW GROWING BABIES

Many of the tests in pregnancy check the growth of your baby. If you have previously had a very small baby, or if you smoke heavily, the midwives and doctors will already be monitoring your pregnancy closely. Blood pressure checks may also pick up signs of trouble. If there is concern about your baby's health, further tests may be carried out and more frequent monitoring of your baby may be recommended.

In the last weeks of pregnancy you may also be asked to keep track of your baby's movements. If you notice your baby's movements becoming less frequent or slowing down, or if they stop, contact your midwife or doctor immediately.

If tests show that your baby is not growing well in the womb, early delivery by induction of labour (see page 97) or Caesarean section (see page 97) may be recommended.

OTHER SYMPTOMS

You should contact your GP if you have a sudden 'acute' illness like acute diarrhoea, vomiting, abdominal pain or a high fever.

HIGH BLOOD PRESSURE AND PRE-ECLAMPSIA

During pregnancy your blood pressure will be checked at every antenatal appointment. This is because a rise in blood pressure can be the first sign of a condition known as pre-eclampsia – often called pregnancy-induced hypertension (PIH) or pre-eclamptic toxaemia (PET) – which can run in families and affects 10% of pregnancies. Your urine will also be checked for protein.

If you do have pre-eclampsia, you will probably feel perfectly well. Some women experience symptoms such as headaches, visual disturbances, swelling and abdominal pain. Pre-eclampsia can still be severe, however, without any symptoms at all. Although most cases are mild and cause no trouble, it can get worse and be serious for both mother and baby. It can cause fits in the mother and affect the baby's growth, and be life-threatening if left untreated. That is why routine antenatal checks are so important.

Pre-eclampsia usually happens towards the end of pregnancy, but problems can occur earlier. Rarely, it can happen after the birth. The earlier in pregnancy it starts, the more severe it is likely to be. If it does get worse, the treatment ranges from rest at home or in hospital, drugs to lower the high blood pressure or, occasionally early delivery of the baby.

VAGINAL BLEEDING

Bleeding from the vagina at any time in pregnancy can be a danger signal. In early pregnancy, bleeding may be a sign of an ectopic pregnancy or a miscarriage (see page 100), although many women who bleed at this time go on to have normal and successful pregnancies. If you have bleeding with pain contact your GP straight away.

Bleeding after about five months may be a sign that the placenta is implanted in the lower part of the uterus (placenta praevia) or that it has started to separate (placental abruption). Both of these can be dangerous for you and the baby, so contact your midwife or doctor immediately.

Bleeding may also be due to the fact that veins in the cervix increase slightly in pregnancy and so it is more likely to bleed, particularly after intercourse. This is known as a cervical erosion and is a normal change that happens in pregnancy. Vaginal infections can also cause a small amount of vaginal bleeding.

Some causes of vaginal bleeding are more serious than others, so it's important to find the cause straight away. The most common sort of bleeding in late pregnancy is the small amount of blood mixed with mucus, known as a 'show'. This is a sign that the cervix is changing and becoming ready for labour to start. It may happen a few days before contractions start or during labour itself. You should always report this to your doctor or midwife as soon as it occurs.

SEVERE ITCHING AND OBSTETRIC CHOLESTASIS

Severe generalised itching, particularly in the last four months of pregnancy, may be the only sign of an uncommon condition called obstetric cholestasis. This is a potentially dangerous liver disorder which seems to run in families, although it can occur without any family history. It is important to contact your doctor if you have troublesome itching because obstetric cholestasis may lead to premature labour, stillbirth or serious health problems for the baby, and to an increased risk of maternal haemorrhage after the delivery.

10 What you need for the baby

T his is a list of essential items you need to get before your baby is born, and some others that you may want to think about. You may be able to borrow some of these items and then pass them on later to another baby. Look out for secondhand equipment too but do check that it is safe. Ask your health visitor if you're in doubt.

NAPPIES

CHOOSING NAPPIES

You can get terry towelling (terries) or disposable. Each has advantages and disadvantages.

Disposable nappies cost more to use but they save time and are useful if washing and drying are a problem where you live.

Terries are cheaper to use, even taking into account the cost of washing them. They are more environmentally friendly but the washing, sterilising and drying do mean more work.

Shaped, washable nappies are also available, often with a Velcro fastening. If you do opt for terry nappies, you'll need two dozen or you'll run out. You also need:

- **nappy pins**
- **nappy liners** – either disposable or cloth, which you can wash and use again
- **plastic pants** – about four pairs, either tie-on or elasticated. Tie-on ones often fit small babies better

- **a bucket with a lid and nappy sterilising powder or liquid** for sterilising nappies.

CHANGING NAPPIES

You'll need:

- **cotton wool** – always choose white, and rolls are cheaper
- **a plastic changing mat** is very useful and convenient but you can make do with a piece of waterproof sheet over an old towel
- **baby lotion or baby wipes** – water is fine and cheap for cleaning your baby's bottom, but lotion or wipes can be convenient, especially when you're out
- **baby barrier cream** to help prevent nappy rash – though the best way to prevent this is by changing and cleaning your baby's bottom well and often
- **a changing bag** to carry all the nappy-changing equipment when you go out. A carrier bag will do but you can get special changing bags that include a changing mat.

81

BATHING

- Any **large, clean bowl** will do as long as it's not metal. Or you can always use the sink, but remember to wrap a towel round the taps for safety.

- You need **baby soap or liquid** which can also be used on babies' hair. Ordinary toilet soap may irritate your baby's skin. It isn't necessary to use baby shampoo.

- **Two towels,** the softer the better. There's no need for special baby towels, unless you want them. Keep the towels for your baby's use only.

SLEEPING

For the first few months, you will need a **crib, a carry cot or a Moses basket.** Your baby just needs somewhere to sleep that is safe and warm and not too far away from you. You also need:

- a **firm mattress** which must fit the cot snugly, without leaving spaces round the edges. The baby could trap his or her head and suffocate. It's best if the mattress has a built–in plastic cover but, if not, you can put a waterproof sheet under the bottom sheet. (Never use thin plastic or a bin liner as your baby could suffocate in the loose folds.)

- **sheets** to cover the mattress – you need at least four because they need to be changed so often. Fitted sheets make life easy but they are quite expensive. You could use pieces of old sheet or pillow cases instead.

- several **light blankets** for safety and warmth.

COT SAFETY

Your baby will spend many hours alone in a cot so make sure it's safe.

- The mattress must fit snugly with no space for a baby's head to get stuck.

- The bars must be smooth, securely fixed and the distance between each bar should be not less than 25 mm and not more than 60 mm so that your baby's head can't be trapped.

- The cot should be sturdy.

- The moving parts should work smoothly and not allow fingers or clothing to become trapped.

- Cot bumpers are not recommended as babies can overheat or become entangled in the fastenings.

- Never leave anything with ties – bibs, clothes, etc. – in the cot in case they get caught around your baby's neck.

- If you're buying a new cot, look for the British Standard mark BS 1753.

See page 117 for more information on reducing the risk of cot death.

This baby is sleeping in the 'feet to foot' position (see page 117). This means that the baby's feet are right at the end of the cot to prevent the baby wriggling under the covers

OUT AND ABOUT

Spend some time looking at what is available for getting your baby about and thinking about what will suit you best before making a choice. You could always ask other mothers what they have found useful.

- **Baby carriers** (also called slings) are attached with straps and your baby is carried in front of you. Most babies like being carried like this because they're close to you and warm. The back part of the carrier must be high enough to support your baby's head. Check that buckles and straps are secure. Older babies who can hold up their heads and whose backs are stronger (at about four months) can be carried in backpacks.

- **Pushchairs** are only suitable for young babies if they have fully reclining seats which let the baby lie flat. Wait until your baby can sit up before using any other pushchair. You should also consider the **weight** of the pushchair if you use public transport.

- **Prams** give your baby a lot of space to sit and lie comfortably although they take up a lot of space and cannot be used on public transport. If you have a car look for a pram which can be dismantled easily. Buy a pram harness at the same time as you will soon need it.

- **Carry cot on wheels** – your baby can sleep in the carry cot for the first few months and the cot can be attached to the frame to go out. It can also be taken in a car.

- **Three-in-one** – this is a carry cot and transporter (set of wheels) that can be converted into a pushchair when your baby outgrows the carry cot.

- **Shopping trays** which fit under the pushchair or pram can be very useful when you're out.

> ### Before buying a pushchair or pram, etc. check that:
>
> - the brakes are sound
>
> - the handles are at the right height for pushing
>
> - the frame is strong enough.

IN THE CAR

If you've got a car, you must have a safety restraint right from the start, even coming home from the hospital. It's very dangerous to carry your baby in your arms, and illegal if you are in the front seat. The best way for your baby to travel is in a rear-facing infant baby restraint (car seat) either on the front or back seat. This is held in place by the adult safety belt. Make sure it's correctly fitted. Do not place a rear-facing infant baby restraint in the front passenger seat if your car is fitted with an air bag.

Do not buy a secondhand car seat as it may have been damaged in an accident. Look for European Standard number R44/03 when you buy.

FEEDING

WASHING BABY CLOTHES

If you use a washing machine, don't use enzyme (bio) powders, as they may irritate your baby's skin. Always rinse very thoroughly. Fabric softener may also cause a skin reaction.

If you're breastfeeding you will probably want **nursing bras.** They should open at the front and have adjustable straps. Cotton is best because it allows air to circulate. If you try on bras at about 36 to 38 weeks they should fit when needed later.

A supply of **breast pads** may also be useful.

If you're going to bottle feed, you will need to get:

- **six bottles** with teats and caps

- **sterilising equipment**

- **a bottle brush**

- **powdered baby milk** – don't buy this too far in advance and remember to check the 'sell by date' on the pack.

CLOTHES FOR THE BABY

Babies grow very quickly. All you need for the first few weeks are enough clothes to make sure that your baby will be warm and clean. You'll probably need:

- **six stretch suits** for both day and night or four stretch suits and two nighties for the night – use socks or bootees with the nightie if it's cold

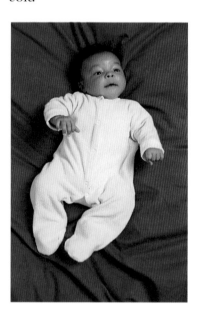

- **two cardigans,** wool rather than nylon, light rather than heavy – several light layers of clothing are best for warmth

- **four vests**

- **a shawl or blanket** to wrap your baby in

- **a woolly hat, mittens, socks or bootees** for going out if the weather is cold – it's better to choose close-knitted patterns for safety

- **a sun hat** for going out if the weather is hot or the sun is bright.

11 Labour and birth

The initial **T**his chapter describes a hospital birth because that is where most people have their babies, but the information will also be useful if you are having a home birth.

GETTING READY FOR THE BIRTH

PACKING FOR HOSPITAL

Pack a bag to take to hospital well in advance. Many hospitals have a printed list of what to pack. If you're having your baby at home your midwife will give you a list of things you should have ready.

You may want to include the following:

- **front-opening nighties** if you're going to breastfeed and an extra one if you're going to wear your nightie, rather than a hospital gown, during labour

- **dressing gown** and **slippers**

- **two or three nursing bras,** or ordinary bras if you're not breastfeeding (remember, your breasts will be much larger than usual)

- about **24 sanitary towels** (super absorbent), not tampons

- **five or six pairs of old pants,** or disposables – you'll probably want to change often to stay fresh

- your **washbag** with toothbrush, hairbrush, flannel, etc.

- **towels** in a dark colour if possible

- **change** or a **phone card** for the hospital payphone

- a **book**, magazines, personal stereo or some knitting, for example, to help you pass the time and relax

- a **loose comfortable outfit** to wear during the day

- a **small bag for labour** with one or two large T-shirts, a sponge or water spray to cool you down, a personal stereo with your favourite music and anything else which you feel will make labour more pleasant for you

- **clothes and nappies** for the baby.

For coming home
Pack loose, easy-to-wear clothes for yourself, baby clothes (including a bonnet), some nappies and a shawl or blanket to wrap the baby in.

TRANSPORT

Work out how you will get to the hospital as it could be at any time of the day or night. If you're planning to go by car, make sure it's running well and that there's always enough petrol in the tank. If a neighbour has said that they will probably be able to take you, make an alternative arrangement just in case they're not in. If you haven't got a car, call an ambulance – try to do so in good time.

HOW TO RECOGNISE WHEN LABOUR STARTS

IF LABOUR STARTS EARLY

Sometimes labour starts early, even as early as 24 weeks. If this happens, get advice immediately from the hospital.

You're unlikely to mistake the signs of labour when the time really comes but, if you're in any doubt, don't hesitate to contact your hospital or midwife and ask for advice.

SIGNS THAT LABOUR IS BEGINNING

Regular contractions
You may have been feeling contractions (Braxton Hicks' contractions) – when your abdomen gets tight and then relaxes – throughout pregnancy. Lately you will have become more aware of them. When they start to come regularly, last more than 30 seconds and begin to feel stronger, labour may have started. Gradually they will become longer, stronger and more frequent.

Other signs of labour
You may or may not also have the following signs:

- **Backache** or that aching, heavy feeling that some women get with their monthly period.

- **A 'show'** – either before labour starts, or early in labour, the plug of mucus in the cervix, which has helped to seal the womb during pregnancy, comes away and comes out of the vagina. This small amount of sticky pink mucus is called a 'show'. You don't lose a lot of blood with a show – just a little, mixed with mucus. If you are losing more blood, it may be a sign that something is wrong. Telephone your hospital or midwife straight away.

- **The waters breaking** – the bag of water in which the baby is floating may break before labour starts. You could keep a sanitary pad (*not* a tampon) handy if you're going out, and put a plastic sheet on the bed. If the waters break before labour starts, you will notice either a slow trickle from your vagina or a sudden gush of water that you can't control. Phone the hospital or your midwife. You will probably be advised to go in at once.

- **Nausea or vomiting.**

- **Diarrhoea.**

PAIN RELIEF IN LABOUR

It's important to learn about all the ways you can relieve pain in labour and how your partner or labour supporter can help you. Ask your midwife or doctor to explain what is available so that you can decide what is best for you. Write down your wishes in your birth plan, but remember you may need to be flexible. Effective pain relief may be advised to assist with delivery.

TYPES OF PAIN RELIEF

Self-help

Using relaxation, breathing, keeping mobile, having a partner to support and massage you, and having confidence in your own body will all help.

'Gas and air' (Entonox)

This is a mixture of oxygen and another gas called nitrous oxide. You breathe it in through a mask which you hold for yourself.

You'll probably have a chance to practise using the mask or mouthpiece if you attend an antenatal class. 'Gas and air' won't remove all the pain but it can help by reducing it and making it easier to bear. Many women like it because it's easy to use and you control it yourself. The gas takes 15 to 20 seconds to work, so you breathe it in just as a contraction begins. There are no harmful side effects for you or the baby, but it can make you feel lightheaded. Some women also find that it makes them feel sick or sleepy or unable to concentrate on what is happening. If this happens you can simply stop using it.

If you try 'gas and air' and find that it does not give you enough pain relief, you can ask for an injection as well.

TENS

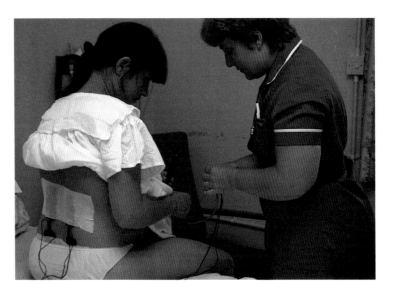

This stands for transcutaneous electrical nerve stimulation and is offered at some hospitals. In others you may need to hire a machine. It lessens the pain for many, but not all, women.

There are no known side effects for either you or the baby and you can move around while using it.

'Gas and air seemed to work for me, provided I used it at the right time. The midwife was really good and helped me with my timing.'

'I didn't want to have any injections or anything, so my midwife told me about TENS. It sounded a bit weird when she told me what it was but, when the time came, it actually did seem to work.'

Electrodes are taped on to your back and connected by wires to a small battery–powered stimulator known as an 'obstetric pulsar'. You hold the pulsar and can give yourself small, safe amounts of current.

It is believed that TENS works by stimulating the body to increase production of its own natural painkillers, called endorphins. It also reduces the number of pain signals that are sent to the brain by the spinal cord. If you're interested in TENS you should learn how to use it in the earlier months of your pregnancy. Ask your midwife or physiotherapist.

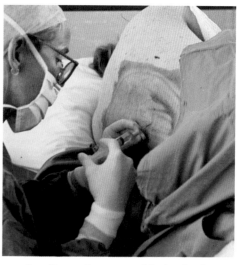

'After the first injection, I felt wonderful, there was no pain and I was on cloud nine. But after the second one, and some gas, I felt confused and out of control, which I think extended the labour.'

Injections

Another form of pain relief is the intramuscular injection of a pain-relieving drug, usually pethidine. It takes about 20 minutes to work and the effects last between two to four hours. It will help you to relax and some women find that this lessens the pain. However, it can make some women feel very 'woozy', sick and forgetful. If it hasn't worn off when you need to push, it can make it difficult. You might prefer to ask for half a dose initially to see how it works for you. If pethidine is given too close to the time of delivery, it may affect the baby's breathing, but if it does an antidote will be given.

'I was really scared about the pain so I chose to have an epidural. It was great – I didn't feel a thing!'

Epidural anaesthesia

An epidural is a special type of local anaesthetic. It numbs the nerves which carry the feelings of pain from the birth canal to the brain. So, for most women, an epidural gives complete pain relief.

An epidural is given by an anaesthetist so, if you think you might want one, check with your midwife beforehand (perhaps when you're discussing your birth plan) about whether an anaesthetist is always available at your hospital.

While you lie on your side, anaesthetic is injected into the space between the bones in your spine through a very thin tube. It takes about 20 minutes to get the tube set up and then another 15 to 20 minutes for it to work. The anaesthetic can then be pumped in continuously or topped up when necessary.

An epidural can be very helpful for those women who are having a long or particularly painful labour or who are becoming very distressed. It takes the pain of labour away for most women and you won't feel so tired afterwards. But there are disadvantages:

- your legs may feel heavy and that sometimes makes women feel rather helpless and unable to get into a comfortable position;

- you may find it difficult to pass water and a small tube called a catheter may need to be put into your bladder to help you;

- you will need to have a drip on your arm to give you fluids and help maintain adequate blood pressure;

- you won't be able to get out of bed during labour and for several hours afterwards;

- your contractions and the baby's heart will need to be monitored by a machine. This means having a belt round your abdomen and possibly a clip attached to your baby's head (see **Fetal heart monitoring**, page 92);

- if you can no longer feel your contractions, the midwife will have to tell you when to push rather than you doing it naturally. Sometimes less anaesthetic is given at the end so that the effect of the epidural wears off and you can push the baby out more effectively;

- some women get backache for some time after having an epidural.

In some hospitals, a mobile or 'walking' epidural is available. The anaesthetist gives a different combination of drugs which allows you to move your legs whilst still providing effective pain relief. Ask if this is available in your hospital.

If you don't want any of these kinds of pain relief, you are free to say so. And if you decide you do want pain relief, ask for it as soon as you feel you need it, without waiting for it to be offered.

ALTERNATIVE METHODS OF PAIN RELIEF

Some mothers want to avoid these methods of pain relief and choose acupuncture, aromatherapy, homeopathy, hypnosis, massage and reflexology. If you would like to use any of these methods, it's important to let the hospital know beforehand.

Discuss the matter with the midwife or doctor. And make sure that the practitioner you use is properly trained and experienced. For advice, contact the Institute for Complementary Medicine (see page 134).

WHAT YOU CAN DO FOR YOURSELF

Fear makes pain worse and everyone feels frightened of what they don't understand or can't control. So learning about labour from antenatal classes, from your doctor or midwife, and from books like this, is an important first step.

- *Learning to relax helps you to remain calmer and birth classes can teach ways of breathing that may help with contractions.*

- *Your position can also make a difference. Some women like to kneel, walk around or rock backwards and forwards. Some like to be massaged, but others hate to be touched.*

- *Feeling in control of what is happening to you is important. You are working with the midwife and she with you, so don't hesitate to ask questions or to ask for anything you want at any time.*

- *Having a partner, friend or relative you can 'lean on', and who can support you during labour certainly helps. It has been shown to reduce the need for pain relief. But if you don't have anyone, don't worry – your midwife will give you the support you need.*

- *And finally, no one can tell you what your labour will feel like in advance. Even if you think you would prefer not to have any pain relief, keep an open mind. In some instances, it could help to make your labour more enjoyable and fulfiling.*

COPING AT THE BEGINNING

KEEPING ACTIVE

Keep active for as long as you feel comfortable. This helps the progress of the birth. Keeping active doesn't mean anything strenuous – just moving normally or walking around.

At night, try getting comfortable and relaxed and perhaps dozing off to sleep. A warm bath or shower may help you to relax. During the day, keep upright and gently active. This helps the baby to move down into the pelvis and the cervix to dilate. It's important to have something light to eat to give you energy, as labour, particularly a first one, may last 12 to 15 hours from the early stages to delivery.

WHEN TO GO INTO HOSPITAL OR GP/MIDWIFE UNIT

If your waters have broken you will probably be advised to go straight in. If your contractions start but your waters have not broken and you live near to the hospital or unit, wait until they are coming regularly, about five minutes apart, lasting about 60 seconds, and they feel so strong that you want to be in hospital. If the journey is likely to take a while, either because of traffic or the distance, or if this is not your first baby, go sooner and make sure you leave plenty of time to get to the hospital. Second and later babies often arrive more quickly. Don't forget to phone the hospital or unit before leaving home and remember your notes or card.

If you're at all uncertain about whether or not it is time for you to go into hospital, always telephone the hospital or unit or your midwife for advice.

HOME/DOMINO DELIVERY

Follow the procedure you have agreed with your midwife during your discussions about the onset of labour.

AT THE HOSPITAL

Going into hospital when you are in labour may be frightening, but attending antenatal classes and visiting the hospital during pregnancy should help. Hospitals and GP/midwife units all vary, so this is just a guide to what is likely to happen. Talk to your midwife about the way things are done at your local hospital or unit and what you would like for your birth. If your wishes can't be met, it's important to understand why (see **Birth plan**, page 34).

YOUR ARRIVAL

If you carry your own notes, take them to the hospital admissions desk. You will be taken to the labour ward, where a midwife will take you to your room and help you change into a hospital gown or a nightdress of your own. Choose an old one that is loose and preferably made of cotton because you'll feel hot during labour and won't want something tight.

EXAMINATION BY THE MIDWIFE

The midwife will ask you about what has been happening so far and will examine you. If you are having a Domino or home delivery, then this examination will take place at home. The midwife will:

- take your pulse, temperature and blood pressure and check your urine;

- feel your abdomen to check the baby's position and record or listen to your baby's heart;

- probably do an internal examination to find out how much your cervix has opened. (Tell her if a contraction is coming so that she can wait until it has passed.) She will then be able to tell you how far your labour has progressed.

These checks will be repeated at intervals throughout your labour – always ask about anything you want to know. If you and your partner have made a birth plan, show your midwife so that she knows your views about your labour and can help you to achieve them. Many women find that they naturally empty their bowels before, or very early, in labour. Very occasionally, if you are constipated, a suppository may be suggested.

DELIVERY ROOMS

Some hospitals may have one or two delivery rooms decorated in a more homely way, with easy chairs and beanbags so that you can easily move around and change your position during labour. Talk to your midwife about this and write your wishes in your birth plan (see page 35).

BATH OR SHOWER

Some hospitals may offer you a bath or shower. A warm bath can be soothing in the early stages of labour. In fact, some women like to spend much of their labour in the bath as a way of easing the pain.

WATER BIRTHS

Some hospitals have birthing pools available (or you may be able to hire one) so that you can labour in water. Many women find that this helps them to relax. If labour progresses normally it may be possible to deliver the baby in the pool. This method is currently being studied, so speak to your midwife and obstetrician about the advantages and disadvantages. You'll need to make arrangements well in advance.

WHAT HAPPENS IN LABOUR

There are three stages to labour. In the first stage the cervix gradually opens up (dilates). In the second stage the baby is pushed down the vagina and is born. In the third stage the placenta comes away from the wall of the womb and is also pushed out of the vagina.

THE FIRST STAGE

The dilatation of the cervix

Contractions at the start of labour help to soften the cervix. Then the cervix will gradually open to about 10 cms. This is wide enough to let the baby out and is called 'fully dilated'. Sometimes the process of softening can take many hours before what midwives refer to as 'established labour'. This is when your cervix has opened (dilated) to at least 3 cms.

If you go into hospital before labour is established, you may be asked if you would prefer to go home again for a while, rather than spending many extra hours in hospital. Once labour is established, the midwife will check again from time to time to see how you are progressing. In a first labour, the time from the start of established labour to full dilatation is between 6 and 12 hours. It is often quicker for later ones.

Towards the end of the first stage, you may feel that you want to push as each contraction comes. At this point, if the midwife isn't already with you, ring for her to come. She will tell you to try not to push until your cervix is fully open and the baby's head can be seen. To help yourself get over the urge to push, try blowing out slowly and gently or, if the urge is too strong, in little

puffs. Some people find this easier lying on their sides, or on their elbows and knees, to reduce the pressure of the baby's head on the cervix.

Fetal heart monitoring

Every baby's heart is monitored throughout labour. The midwife is watching for any marked change in the heart rate which could be a sign that the baby is distressed and that action should be taken in order to speed delivery. There are different ways of monitoring the baby's heartbeat.

● Your midwife may listen to the baby's heart intermittently with a hand-held ultrasound monitor (often called a Sonicaid). This method allows you to be free to move around in labour if you wish.

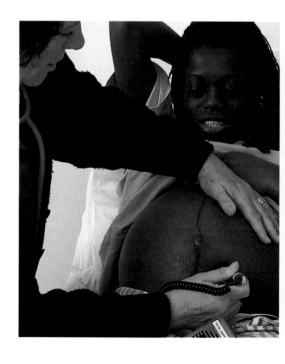

● The heartbeat and contractions may also be followed electronically through a monitor linked to a machine called a CTG. The monitor will be strapped on a belt to your tummy.

Sometimes it may be suggested that a clip is put on the baby's head so that its heart can be monitored more exactly. The clip is put on during a vaginal examination and the waters are broken if they have not already done so. Ask your midwife or doctor to explain why they feel the clip is necessary for your baby. Throughout labour the heartbeat will be followed by a bleep from the machine and a print out. You cannot easily move around. Some machines use tiny transmitters which allow you to be more mobile. Ask if this is available.

A drip may be used to speed up labour.

Speeding up labour

If your labour is slow, your doctor may recommend acceleration to get things moving. You should be given a clear explanation of why this is proposed. To start with your waters will be broken (if this has not already happened) during a vaginal examination. This is often enough to get things moving. If not, you may be offered a drip containing a hormone which will encourage contractions. If you have a drip, the hormone will be fed into a vein in your arm.

The baby's birth

This stage begins when the cervix is fully dilated and lasts until the birth of the baby. Your body will tell you to push. Listen to your midwife who will guide you.

Position

Find the position that you prefer and which will make labour easier for you. You might want to remain in bed with your back propped up with pillows, or stand, sit, kneel or squat (squatting will take practice if you are not used to it). If you are very tired, you might be more comfortable lying on your side rather than your back. This is also a better position for your baby.

If you've suffered from backache in labour, kneeling on all fours might be helpful. It's up to you. Try out some of these positions at antenatal classes or at home to find out which are the most comfortable for you. Ask the midwife to help you.

Pushing

You can now start to push each time you have a contraction. Your body will probably tell you how. If not, take two deep breaths as the contractions start and push down.

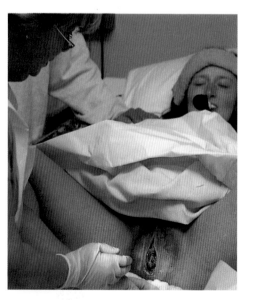

Take another breath when you need to. Give several pushes until the contraction ends. As you push, try to let yourself 'open up' below. After each contraction, rest and get up strength for the next one. This stage is hard work but your midwife will help you all the time, telling you what to do and encouraging you. Your companion can also give you lots of support. Ask your midwife to tell you what is happening. This stage may take an hour or more, so it helps to know how you're doing.

The birth

As the baby's head moves into the vaginal opening you can put your hand down to feel it, or look at it in a mirror. When about half the head can be seen, the midwife will tell you to stop pushing, to push very gently, or to puff a couple of quick short breaths blowing out through your mouth. This is so that your baby's head can be born slowly, giving the skin and muscles of the perineum (the area between your vagina and back passage) time to stretch without tearing.

Sometimes the skin of the perineum won't stretch enough and may tear. Or there may be an urgency to hurry the birth because the baby is getting short of oxygen. The midwife or doctor will then ask

Once the baby's head is born, the body usually follows quite quickly and easily with one more push.

You can have your baby lifted straight on to you before the cord is cut.

Your baby may be born still covered with some of the white, greasy vernix which acts as a protection in the womb.

your permission to give you a local anaesthetic and cut the skin to make the opening bigger. This is called an episiotomy. Afterwards the cut or tear is stitched up again and heals. Once your baby's head is born, most of the hard work is over. With one more gentle push the body is born quite quickly and easily. You can ask to have the baby lifted straight onto you before the cord is cut, so that you can feel and be close to each other immediately. Then the cord is clamped and cut, the baby is dried to prevent him or her from becoming cold, and you'll be able to hold and cuddle your baby properly. Your baby may be quite messy, with some of your blood and perhaps some of the white, greasy vernix which acts as a protection in the womb still on the skin. If you prefer, you can ask the midwife to wipe your baby and wrap him or her in a blanket before your cuddle.

Sometimes some mucus has to be cleared out of a baby's nose and mouth or some oxygen given to get breathing underway. Your baby won't be kept away from you any longer than necessary.

THE THIRD STAGE

The placenta

After your baby is born, more contractions will push out the placenta. This stage can take between 20 minutes and an hour but your midwife will usually give you an injection in your thigh, just as the baby is born, which will speed it up.

The injection contains a drug called Syntometrine which makes the womb contract and so helps prevent the heavy bleeding which some women may experience without it. You may prefer not to have the injection at first, but to wait and see if it is necessary. You should discuss this in advance with your midwife and make a note on your birth plan.

95

'All I wanted afterwards was to go to sleep.'

'I kept looking at him and thinking, "I've actually got one! He's mine! I've done it at last!"'

'It was like being drunk, I felt so special, so full of myself and what I'd done.'

A paediatrician may check your baby straight after delivery.

If you're breastfeeding, let your baby suckle as soon after birth as possible. Babies do suck this soon, although maybe just for a short time, or they may just like to feel the nipple in the mouth. It helps with breastfeeding later on and it also helps your womb to contract.

AFTERWARDS

If you've had a deep tear or an episiotomy, it will be sewn up. If you have had an epidural you will not feel this. Otherwise you should be offered a local anaesthetic injection. If it is sore during this repair, then say so; it is the only way that the midwife or doctor will know that they are hurting you. Small tears and grazes are often left to heal without stitches because they frequently heal better this way.

Your baby will be examined, weighed and possibly measured and given a band with your name on it. The midwife will then help you to wash and freshen up. Then you should have some time alone with your baby and your partner, just to be together quietly and meet your new baby properly. If you find this doesn't happen and you would like some time alone, ask for it.

SPECIAL CASES

LABOUR THAT STARTS TOO EARLY (PREMATURE LABOUR)

About one baby in every ten will be born before the 37th week of pregnancy. In most cases labour starts by itself, either with contractions or with the sudden breaking of the waters or a show (see page 86). About one early baby in three is induced (see page 90) or delivered by Caesarean section (see pages 90-91) because doctors feel that early delivery is necessary for your own or the baby's safety.

If your baby is likely to be delivered early, you will be admitted to a hospital with specialist facilities for premature babies. Not all hospitals have facilities for the care of very premature babies, so it may be necessary to transfer you and your baby to another unit, either before delivery or immediately afterwards. If contractions start well before you are due, the doctors may be able to use drugs to stop your contractions temporarily. You will probably be advised to have injections of steroids that will help to mature your baby's lungs so that he or she is better able to breathe after the birth. This treatment takes about 24 hours to work.

If you have any reason to think that your labour may be starting early, get in touch with your hospital or midwife at once so that arrangements can be made.

BABIES BORN LATE

Pregnancy normally lasts about 40 weeks, that is 280 days from the first day of your last period. Most women will go into labour within two weeks either side of this date. If your labour does not start, the doctor will want to keep a careful check on your baby's health. This is often referred to as 'monitoring'. If there is any evidence that your baby is not doing well, or if you are overdue by two weeks, the doctor will suggest that labour is started artificially.

INDUCTION

Sometimes labour must be started artificially. This is called induction. Labour may be induced if there is any sort of risk to the mother's or baby's health – for example, if the mother has high blood pressure or if the baby is failing to grow and thrive. Induction is always planned in advance, so you will be able to talk over the advantages and disadvantages with your doctor and midwife and find out why it is thought suitable in your particular case.

Contractions can be started by inserting a pessary or gel into the vagina, or by a hormone drip in the arm. Sometimes both are used. Induction of labour may take a while, particularly if the neck of the womb (cervix) needs to be softened with pessaries or gels. Once labour starts it should proceed normally.

FORCEPS DELIVERY OR VACUUM EXTRACTION

If the baby needs to be helped out of the vagina – perhaps because the contractions aren't strong enough, because the baby has got into an awkward position or is becoming distressed, or because you have become too exhausted – then forceps or vacuum extraction (sometimes called Ventouse) will be used.

A local anaesthetic will usually be given to numb the birth canal, if you haven't already had an epidural or spinal anaesthetic.

Forceps are placed round the baby's head by an obstetrician and with gentle firm pulling the baby can be born. With vacuum delivery, a shallow rubber or metal cap is fitted to the baby's head by suction. You can help by pushing when the obstetrician asks you to. Sometimes you will find red marks on your baby's head where the forceps have been or a swelling from the vacuum. They will soon fade.

An episiotomy (see page 95) is nearly always needed for a forceps delivery.

Your partner or companion should be able to stay with you if you wish.

CAESAREAN SECTION

The baby is delivered by cutting through the abdomen and then into the womb. The cut is usually done crossways and low down, just below the bikini line. It is usually hidden when your pubic hair grows back again.

A Caesarean section may be 'elective' (that is, planned in advance) or 'emergency'. An elective Caesarean may be recommended if

HEPATITIS B

If you have hepatitis B when you give birth, your baby will be immunised to stop him or her being infected.

'I wasn't elated or anything like that. I think it had all been too much like hard work to feel much after.'

'I was relieved. I was delighted about the baby, but I was more relieved than anything – that it was over, and we'd come through, and everything was fine'.

(A FATHER)

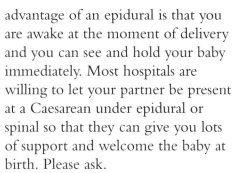

advantage of an epidural is that you are awake at the moment of delivery and you can see and hold your baby immediately. Most hospitals are willing to let your partner be present at a Caesarean under epidural or spinal so that they can give you lots of support and welcome the baby at birth. Please ask.

labour is judged to be dangerous for you or the baby. An emergency Caesarean may be necessary if complications develop and delivery needs to be quick. This may be before or during labour. Sometimes the cervix does not dilate fully during labour and an emergency Caesarean will be suggested but, providing you and the baby are well, there is no need to proceed with great haste.

Whenever a Caesarean is suggested, your doctor should explain why it is necessary and any possible side effects. Do not hesitate to ask questions.

Where possible, the operation is performed under epidural anaesthesia (see page 88) or the similar spinal anaesthetic. A general anaesthetic is sometimes used, particularly when the baby needs to be delivered very quickly or if there are technical problems, but this increases the risks for you and the baby. This is why epidural and spinal anaesthetics are recommended.

If you have an epidural, you will be awake throughout the operation but you won't feel pain, just some tugging and pulling and wetness when the waters break. A screen will be put across your chest so that you cannot see what is being done. The doctors will talk to you and let you know what is happening.

The operation is safe and takes about 30 to 40 minutes. One

After a Caesarean you will be uncomfortable for a few days, as you would expect to be after any major surgery. It will be difficult to sit up or stand up straight and it will hurt to laugh. You will have to stay in hospital a bit longer, about five to seven days, but this will depend on your condition. You will also have to take it easy once you are home and you will need help. You shouldn't lift anything heavy or drive a car for six weeks. Your doctor or midwife will advise you on how much you can do. Postnatal exercises are especially important after a Caesarean to get your muscles working again, but take things at a gentle pace. The midwife or hospital physiotherapist will tell you when you should begin them. You can also contact the Caesarean Support Network for information and support (see page 134).

BREECH BIRTH

A breech birth is when a baby is born bottom first. This is often considered a reason for Caesarean delivery though it is possible for a baby to be born this way quite normally. More care is needed to avoid damage to the baby, especially when delivering the head, and forceps are quite often used (see page 97). An epidural is often recommended. In some units you may be offered the option of an external cephalic version (ECV). The baby is turned into the usual head down position (cephalic) by pressing on the woman's tummy.

TWINS

If you are expecting twins, labour may start early because the womb becomes very stretched with two babies. More people will usually be present at the birth – for example, a midwife, an obstetrician, and usually two paediatricians, one for each baby.

The process of labour is the same but the babies will be closely monitored, usually by using an electronic monitor (see page 93). You will be given a drip in case it is needed later and an epidural will often be recommended. Once the first baby has been born, the midwife or doctor will check the position of the second by feeling your abdomen and doing a vaginal examination. If the second baby is in a good position to be born, the waters surrounding the baby will be broken and the second baby should be born very soon after the first because the cervix is already fully dilated. If contractions stop after the first birth, hormones will be added to the drip to restart them.

If you're expecting twins or more babies, you might like to contact the Twins and Multiple Births Association (TAMBA) for advice and support (see page 135).

WHAT YOUR COMPANION CAN DO

Whoever your labour partner is – the baby's father, a close friend, or a relative – there are quite a few practical things that he or she can do to help you, although probably none of them are as important as just being with you. You can't know in advance what your labour is going to be like or how each of you will cope. But there are many ways in which a partner can help.

Your labour partner can:

- keep you company and help pass the time in the early stages;

- hold your hand, wipe your face, give you sips of water, massage your back and shoulders, help you move about or change position, or anything else that helps and comforts you as your labour progresses and your contractions get stronger;

- remind you how to use relaxation and breathing techniques, perhaps breathing with you if it helps;

- support your decisions about, for example, pain relief;

- help you make it clear to the midwife or doctor what help you need – and the other way round. This can help you to feel much more in control of the situation;

- as your baby is born, tell you what is happening, because you can't see what is going on for yourself.

For very many couples, being together during labour and welcoming their baby together is an experience that they can't begin to put into words. And many fathers who have seen their baby born and who have played a part themselves say they feel much closer to the child from the very start.

12 When pregnancy goes wrong

Unfortunately, not all pregnancies end well. For a few, pregnancy ends with a miscarriage or with the death of the baby. This chapter describes some of the things that can go wrong. If your pregnancy ends in this way, then you will need both information and support. Talk to the people close to you about how you feel and to your doctor, midwife or health visitor about what has happened and why. Sometimes it is easier to talk to someone outside your immediate circle. Organisations offering information and support are listed on page 134.

ECTOPIC PREGNANCY

After fertilisation the egg should move down into the womb to develop. Sometimes it gets stuck in the fallopian tube and begins to grow there. This is called an 'ectopic' or 'tubal' pregnancy. The fertilised egg can't develop properly and has to be removed in an operation.

A common cause of an ectopic pregnancy is some sort of blockage in the fallopian tube, possibly as a result of an infection. Warning signs start soon after a missed period. They are a severe pain on one side, low down in the abdomen, vaginal bleeding or brown discharge, and sometimes feeling faint, and women should see their doctor immediately.

Talk to your doctor to find out why it happened and whether your chances of conceiving a baby have been affected. One organisation which can offer support is called Child (see page 134).

MISCARRIAGE

If a pregnancy ends in the first six months it is known as a miscarriage. Miscarriages are quite common in the first three months of pregnancy. Probably at least one in six clinically recognised pregnancies ends this way. At this stage a miscarriage usually happens because there is something wrong with the baby. A later miscarriage may be due to the placenta not developing or working properly, or the cervix being weak and opening too early in the pregnancy.

An early miscarriage can be rather like a period, with bleeding and a similar sort of aching pain, maybe occurring on and off, happening at the time when a period would have been due. With a later miscarriage, bleeding is likely to be accompanied by pains that feel more like the pains that come with labour.

If you bleed or begin to have pains, you should contact the person who is giving you antenatal care, either at the hospital or your GP's surgery. You may be told to lie down quietly or to come into hospital immediately. Sometimes the bleeding stops by itself and your pregnancy will carry on quite normally. But if a miscarriage is going to happen, there is very little that anyone can do to stop it.

After a miscarriage, you may have a 'D and C' (that is, dilation and curettage) to empty the womb. This is done under anaesthetic. The cervix is gently widened and the lining of the womb scraped or sucked away. The cervix narrows again afterwards.

AFTERWARDS

One miscarriage will not affect your chances of having a baby in the future. Even after three miscarriages you still stand a good chance of carrying a baby to term. If you have three or more miscarriages, you should be referred for further investigations. In some cases, all investigations will be normal and no precise cause found.

A miscarriage can be very difficult to come to terms with. You may feel disappointed, angry, or even guilty, wondering what you did wrong. Some people fear that the miscarriage may have been caused by making love, though this is extremely unlikely. In fact, whatever the cause, it is very rarely anyone's fault.

You will almost certainly feel a sense of loss. You need time to grieve over the lost baby just as you would over the death of anyone close to you, especially if the miscarriage has happened later in pregnancy. Many people find it helps to have something to remember their baby by. In early pregnancy you might be able to have a picture of a scan. After about four months you could ask for a photograph of the baby. If your miscarriage is very late you may be able to see and hold your baby, if you wish, as well as having a photograph. Talking also helps. Talk about your feelings with your partner and those close to you. The Miscarriage Association (see page 135) can give you information and put you in touch with other women who have experienced a miscarriage.

TERMINATION

If tests show that your baby has a serious abnormality you may consider whether or not to end your pregnancy (see page 53). It is important to find out as much information as you can from the doctor about the particular condition and how it may affect your baby, so that you can make a decision that is right for you and your family.

You will probably be very shocked when you are first told the diagnosis by the consultant and may not be able to take very much in. You may need to go back and talk again, preferably accompanied by your partner or someone close to you. You will also need to spend time talking things through with your partner or with others close to you.

An early termination, before 12 to 14 weeks, will usually be done under a general anaesthetic. For a later termination you will probably go through labour as this is usually the safest way for you. You may wish to think beforehand about whether you want to see and perhaps even hold your baby and give your baby a name. It can make the baby more real for you and your family and help you to grieve. If you don't wish to see your baby, it's still a good idea to ask hospital staff to take a photograph for you. You may find this comforting at a later date.

You may find your feelings quite hard to cope with after a termination, whether it has been in early or late pregnancy. It will help to talk about them. If you would like to talk to people who have undergone a similar experience you can contact SATFA (Support Around Termination For Abnormality) (see page 135).

LOSING A BABY

In the UK about 4000 babies every year are stillborn – the baby is already dead when it is born. About the same number die soon after birth. Often the causes of these deaths are not known.

If you lose a baby like this, you are likely to feel very shocked. But you and your partner may find it comforting to see and hold your baby and give your baby a name. You may also like to have a photograph of your baby and to keep some mementos such as a lock of hair or the shawl the baby was wrapped in. All this can help you and your family to remember your baby as a real person and can, in time, help in coming to terms with your loss. Many hospitals have a bereavement counsellor who will help you to find the best way for you and your partner to cope with your loss.

One of the first questions you are likely to ask is why your baby died. The doctors and midwives may not know. A post mortem examination is usually advised and this may help to find out, although it doesn't always provide the answer. Most hospitals will offer you an appointment with the consultant who can explain to you what is known. If you are not offered an appointment, you can ask for one.

It may also help to talk about your feelings to other parents who have lost a baby in a similar way. SANDS (the Stillbirth and Neonatal Death Society) is an organisation that can put you in touch with other parents who can offer friendly help (see page 135).

You may well want to arrange a cremation, funeral or service. You should be able to do so. If the baby was lost after 24 weeks, the loss will need to be officially registered as either a death or a stillbirth. If you want to arrange a funeral or cremation and your baby was lost before 24 weeks, you will need a certificate from the hospital. Talk to your midwife or doctor about what you want to do and to find out what arrangements are available locally. You could also consult the hospital chaplain or rabbi or your own religious adviser.

13 The first days with your new baby

In the first few days after the birth, you and your baby are beginning to get to know each other. Don't feel you have to make a great effort. Just have your baby close to you as much as you can.

Partners also need plenty of opportunity to handle the baby and feel close. Many fathers feel a little left out, especially if they have to leave you and the baby in hospital and return to an empty home. They may need support and encouragement to get involved, but the more you can both hold and cuddle your baby the more confident you'll all feel.

YOU

You may feel tired for the first few days, so make sure you get plenty of rest. Even just walking and moving about can seem like hard work. If you've had stitches they'll feel sore and you may feel worried about going to the toilet.

Once your breasts start to fill with milk they may feel uncomfortable or painful for a day or so. If you're breastfeeding, it will help to feed your baby as often as he or she needs (see page 62). You might also like to apply a warm cloth just before a feed to help relieve the engorgement. If you intend to bottle feed from the start you needn't do anything but, on the third or fourth day, your breasts may be tender as the milk is still being produced. Wearing a firm, supportive bra may help. Speak to your midwife if you are very uncomfortable.

For a lot of mothers the excitement and the pleasure of the new baby far outweigh any problems. But some do begin to feel low (see page 113) or rather depressed, especially if they are very tired or feel that they are not making any progress or can't look after their baby as they would like.

Giving birth is an emotional and tiring experience and your hormones change dramatically in the first few days. Some women feel rather weepy around the third day, especially if the labour was difficult, or if they are very tired or have other worries. This is known as the 'baby blues'. Some women worry because they don't love their baby immediately but, as with any relationship, it's not always love at first sight. You may just need to give yourself time – you can still care for your baby and provide all the warmth and security he or she needs.

'I don't think I'll ever forget those first few days. Feeling so happy. Though I don't know why. I couldn't sleep, the ward was so noisy. I was sore. I couldn't move about very well. I missed Alan and home. But I felt happier than I can ever begin to say.'

'I couldn't believe it. I'd never been much of a one for babies. And Dean wasn't even a pretty baby, not at first. Very spotty and blotchy. But he was perfect to me. He bowled me over.'

'I felt awful. I was so tired, on top of everything else. But there was one thing about it. Bob got to know the baby much better than he would have done if I'd been more on top. He was holding her and cuddling her right from the start.'

'I had a lovely rest. No work. Meals provided. Just me and the baby, being together. It was lovely.'

'I'd never been so tired! I spent all my time rushing between the hospital and the flat, catching up on sleep when I could. And the phone never stopped ringing.'

(A FATHER)

'It all seemed a bit of an anti-climax after the birth and everything, and it felt really funny going home to an empty house. But I knew I could see them whenever I wanted to, so it wasn't so bad.'

(A FATHER)

BEING IN HOSPITAL

If you have your baby in hospital, you'll probably be moved to the postnatal ward after the birth to be with other mothers who have also had their babies. Some mothers enjoy their stay in hospital and find it restful and easy. Others find it tiring and rather stressful. It depends on how you're feeling, whether you like the company of other mothers or miss your privacy, and on how the ward is organised. In any case, your stay in hospital, if your delivery is uncomplicated, is likely to be short.

It helps if you've discussed your postnatal care with your midwife during pregnancy so you know what to expect. Any preferences can then be recorded on your birth plan (see page 35) so that staff on the postnatal ward will be aware of your wishes.

You're likely to need quite a lot of help and advice with your first baby. The midwives are there to guide and support you as well as checking that you are recovering from the birth. Don't hesitate to ask for help if you need it. If you do have a problem with the way things are organised in hospital, talk it over with one of the staff. Perhaps a change can be made.

If all is going well with both you and the baby, then most hospitals will probably give you the option of going home after 48 hours or even earlier, even if it's your first baby.

The community midwife will visit you at home and continue to help you to care for yourself and your baby. You will need to make sure that your partner or someone else can be there to help you at home and do the cooking and housework.

STITCHES

If you've had stitches, bathing the area often will help healing. Use a bath, shower or cotton wool and plain warm water. After bathing, dry the vulva carefully. Pelvic floor exercises can also help healing (see page 14). If the stitches are sore and uncomfortable, tell your midwife as she may be able to recommend treatment. Painkilling tablets will also help. If there is swelling and bruising, it may be possible to have some ultrasound treatment from the physiotherapist. In any case, remember to sit down gently and lie on your side rather than your back to start with.

The thought of passing urine can be a bit frightening at first because of the soreness and because you can't seem to feel what you are doing. Sometimes it's easier to pass urine while sitting in a bowl of water or a warm bath. The water dilutes the urine so that it doesn't sting. If you really find it impossible to pass urine, tell your midwife. Also drink lots of water to dilute the urine.

You probably won't need to open your bowels for a few days after the birth but it's important not to let yourself become constipated. Eat fresh fruit, vegetables, salad and brown bread, and drink plenty of water. This should mean that when you do open your bowels you will pass a stool more easily. Whatever it may feel like, it's very unlikely that you will break the stitches or open up the cut or tear again, but it might feel better if you hold a pad of clean tissue over the stitches when you are trying to pass a stool. Avoid straining for the first few days. Sometimes stitches have to be taken out but usually they just dissolve after a week or so, by which time the cut or tear will have healed.

PILES

Piles (see page 77) are very common after delivery but they usually disappear within a few days. Eat plenty of fresh fruit, vegetables, salad, brown bread and wholegrain cereals, and drink plenty of water. This should make it easier and less painful when you pass a stool. Try not to push or strain as this will make the piles worse. Let the midwife know if you feel very uncomfortable. She will be able to give you an ointment to soothe them.

BLEEDING

After the birth you will lose blood and discharge from the vagina. The loss will probably be quite heavy at first which is why you will need super absorbent sanitary towels. Do **not** use tampons until after your postnatal check since they can cause infections in the early weeks after the birth. During breastfeeds you may notice that the discharge is more red or heavier. You may also have 'after pains'. These are both because feeding causes the womb to contract. They are a good sign that everything inside you is going back to normal. Bleeding often becomes heavier around seven to ten days after delivery but, if you find you are losing blood in large clots, you should save these towels to show the midwife as you may need some treatment. Gradually, the discharge will become a brownish colour and may continue for some weeks, getting less and less.

If you're breastfeeding you may not have another period until you stop feeding or even for some weeks or months after that. If you are not breastfeeding, your first period might start as early as a month after the birth. But it could be much later. You can become pregnant before your period starts even if you are breastfeeding, so make sure you decide on a reliable form of contraception before you and your partner make love again (see page 113).

YOUR SHAPE

Your breasts will be larger at first and while you are breastfeeding regularly. You need to wear a supportive nursing bra if you are breastfeeding. If you are not breastfeeding your breasts will reduce in size in a week or so.

Your abdomen will seem quite baggy after delivery. Despite having delivered your baby plus the placenta and a lot of fluid, you will still be quite a lot bigger than you were before pregnancy. This is partly because your muscles have stretched. If you eat a balanced diet and exercise, your shape should soon return to normal. Breastfeeding helps because it makes the womb contract. Sometimes, because this is happening, you may feel a quite painful twinge in your abdomen or period-type pain while you are feeding. Breastfeeding also uses up more calories so it can help you to lose some of the weight gained in pregnancy. Some women do not return to their normal weight until after they have finished breastfeeding.

Postnatal exercises (see page 111) will help to tone up the muscles of your pelvic floor and tummy and help you find your waist again! They will also get you moving and feeling generally fitter. You may be able to attend a postnatal exercise class while you are in hospital and afterwards. Ask your midwife or physiotherapist.

It is quite common after having a baby to find it difficult to control your bladder if you laugh, or move suddenly, and to leak some water. Pelvic floor exercises (see page 14) will help with this. If the problem persists after three months, see your doctor who may refer you to a physiotherapist.

'That first week was nothing but problems. One thing after another, first me and then the baby. Everybody was very helpful, but it was still a week or two before I got sorted out.'

CONTRACEPTION

(see also page 113)
Before you leave hospital, a midwife or doctor will probably talk to you about contraception. If this doesn't happen, you may want to ask. Although it may seem very early to be thinking about making love again, it can be easier to sort out any questions about contraception while you are in hospital rather than later on.

RUBELLA

If you were not immune to rubella (German measles) when tested early in your pregnancy, you will probably be offered immunisation before you leave hospital or shortly afterwards by your GP. If this doesn't happen, ask. This is a good opportunity to get it done. You should not get pregnant again for one month after the injection.

RHESUS NEGATIVE MOTHERS

If your blood group is rhesus negative and your partner's is rhesus positive, blood samples will be taken after delivery to see whether your baby is rhesus positive and whether you need an injection to protect your next baby from anaemia. If so, the injection should be given within 72 hours of delivery. Check with one of the doctors or midwives what should happen in your particular case.

YOUR BABY

Soon after birth you'll be able to look properly at your baby and notice every detail – the colour and texture of the hair – the shape of the hands and feet, and the different expressions on your baby's face. If you notice anything that worries you, however small, ask your doctor or midwife. Your baby will be examined by a doctor to make sure everything is all right. It's a good time to ask any questions you might have.

THE NAVEL

Shortly after birth the midwife will clamp the umbilical cord close to your baby's navel with a plastic clip. She then cuts the cord, leaving a small bit of cord with the clamp attached. The cord will take about a week to dry out and drop off. Keep the navel clean and dry until this happens. The midwife will show you how. If you notice any bleeding from the navel, tell your midwife, health visitor or doctor.

VITAMIN K

We all need vitamin K to make our blood clot properly so that we won't bleed too easily. Some newborn babies have too little vitamin K. Although this is rare, it can cause them to bleed dangerously into the brain. To prevent this, you should be offered vitamin K which will be given to your baby. We don't yet know which is the safest way of giving vitamin K, whether by injection or by mouth. Your doctor or midwife will help you to choose the method you prefer.

THE FONTANELLE

On the top of your baby's head near the front, is a diamond-shaped patch where the skull bones haven't yet fused together. This is called the fontenelle. It will probably be a year or more before the bones close over it. You may notice it moving as your baby breathes. You needn't worry about touching it. There is a tough layer of membrane under the skin.

BUMPS AND BRUISES

It's quite common for a newborn baby to have some swelling and bruises on the head, and perhaps to have bloodshot eyes. This is just the result of the squeezing and pushing that is part of being born and will soon disappear. But if you are at all worried, you can always ask your midwife.

BIRTHMARKS AND SPOTS

Once you begin to look closely at your baby, you'll probably find a variety of little marks and spots, mainly on the head and face, or sometimes larger marks. Most of them will go away eventually. Ask the doctor who examines your baby if they will disappear completely. Most common are the little pink or red marks some people call 'stork bites'. These V–shaped marks on the forehead and upper eyelids gradually fade, though it may be some months before they disappear. Marks on the nape of the neck can go on much longer, but they will be covered by hair.

Strawberry marks are quite common. They are dark red and slightly raised. They sometimes appear a few days after birth and gradually get bigger. They may take a while to go away, but usually they will go away eventually.

Spots and rashes are very common in newborn babies and may come and go. But if you also notice a change in your baby's behaviour, for example if your baby is not feeding properly or is very sleepy or very irritable, you should tell your doctor or midwife immediately.

BREASTS AND GENITALS

Quite often a newborn baby's breasts are a little swollen and ooze some milk, whether the baby is a boy or a girl. Girls also sometimes bleed a bit or have a white, cloudy discharge from the vagina. All this is as a result of hormones passing from the mother to the baby before birth and is no cause for concern. The genitals of male and female newborn babies often appear rather swollen but will look in proportion with their bodies in a few weeks.

JAUNDICE

On about the third day after birth, some babies develop a yellow colour to their skin and a yellowness in the whites of their eyes because of mild jaundice. This usually fades within ten days or so. But a baby who becomes badly jaundiced may need treatment (see page 109).

WHAT A NEWBORN BABY CAN DO

There is one important skill that babies don't have to learn. They are born knowing how to suck. During the first few days they learn to co-ordinate their sucking and their breathing.

Newborn babies also automatically turn towards a nipple or teat if it is brushed against one cheek and they will open their mouths if their upper lip is stroked. They can also grasp things (like your finger) with either hands or feet and they will make stepping movements if they are held upright on a flat surface. All these automatic responses except sucking, are lost within a few months, and your baby will begin to make controlled movements instead.

Newborn babies can use all their senses. They will look at people and things, especially if they are near, and particularly at people's faces. They will enjoy gentle touch, and the sound of a soothing voice and they will react to bright light and noise. Very soon they will also know their mother's special smell.

Who's the most beautiful baby?

14 Babies who need special care

Some babies need special care in hospital, sometimes on the ordinary postnatal ward and sometimes in a Neonatal Unit (NNU), also known as a Special Care Baby Unit (SCBU) or Neonatal Intensive Care Unit (NICU). Babies who may need special care include:

- babies who are born early. Babies born earlier than 34 weeks may need extra help breathing, feeding and keeping warm. The earlier they are born the more help they are likely to need;

- babies who are very small or who have life-threatening conditions, usually affecting their breathing, heart and circulation;

- babies born to diabetic mothers, or babies where the delivery has been very difficult, may need to be kept under close observation for a time;

- babies with very marked jaundice;

- babies awaiting or recovering from complex surgery.

CONTACT WITH YOUR BABY

All babies need cuddling and touching, whether they are in the ward close by you or in an NNU. If your baby is in an NNU, you and your partner should try to be with your baby as much as possible. Encourage other members of your family to visit too, to get to know the baby, if this is possible. When you first go into the NNU you may be put off by all the machines and apparatus. Ask the nurse to explain what everything is for and to show you how to handle your baby.

FEEDING

Feeding is especially important for premature babies. Those who get some of their mother's milk do better, so think seriously about breastfeeding. Even if you can't stay with your baby all the time, you can express milk for the nurses to give while you are away. Some small babies can't suck properly at first and are fed by a fine tube which is passed through the nose or mouth into the stomach. You and your partner can still touch and probably hold your baby. The tube isn't painful, so you needn't worry about it being in the way or hurting your baby.

INCUBATORS

Babies who are very tiny are nursed in incubators rather than cots to keep them warm. But you can still have a lot of contact with your baby. Some incubators have open tops but, if not, you can put your hands through the holes in the side of the incubator to stroke and touch your baby. You can talk to your baby too. This is important for both of you. You may be asked to wear a gown and mask. Carefully wash and thoroughly dry your hands before touching your baby.

NEWBORN BABIES WITH JAUNDICE

Jaundice in newborn babies is common because their livers are immature. Severely jaundiced babies may be treated by phototherapy. The baby is undressed and put under a very bright light, usually with a soft mask over the eyes. It may be possible for your baby to have phototherapy by your bed so that you don't have to be separated. This treatment may continue for several days, with breaks for feeds, before the jaundice clears up. In some cases, if the jaundice gets worse, an exchange transfusion of blood may be needed. Some babies have jaundice because of liver disease and need different treatment. A blood test before phototherapy is started checks for liver disease.

BABIES WITH JAUNDICE AFTER TWO WEEKS

Many babies are jaundiced for up to two weeks following birth. This is common in breastfed babies and usually it's normal and does no harm. It is not a reason to stop breastfeeding. But it's important to ensure that all is well if your baby is still jaundiced **after** two weeks. You should see your doctor within a day or two. This is particularly important if your baby's stools are pale. A simple urine test will distinguish between 'breast milk' jaundice, which will resolve itself, or jaundice which may need urgent treatment.

A BABY WITH DISABILITIES

If your baby is disabled in some way, you will be coping with a muddle of different feelings – love mixed with fear, pity mixed with anger. You will also need to cope with the feelings of others – your partner, relations and friends – as they come to terms with the fact that your baby is different. More than anything else at this time you will need to have a person or people to whom you can talk about how you feel and information about your baby's immediate and future prospects.

There are a number of people to whom you can turn for help – your own GP, a paediatrician at your hospital, or your health visitor. Once you are at home you can contact your social services department for information about local voluntary or statutory organisations. On page 134 you will find a list of organisations which can offer help and advice. Many are self-help groups run by parents. Talking to other parents with similar experiences can often be the most effective help.

On page 134

WORRIES AND EXPLANATIONS

Always ask about the treatment your baby is being given and why, if it's not explained to you. It is important that you understand what is happening so that you can work together with hospital staff to ensure that your baby receives the best possible care. It is natural to feel anxious if your baby is having special care. Talk over any fears or worries with the staff caring for your baby. The consultant paediatrician will probably arrange to see you, but you can also ask for an appointment if you wish. The hospital social worker may be able to help with practical problems.

15 The early weeks: you

Going home from hospital can be very exciting, but you may feel nervous too without the hospital staff on call to help you. The more you handle your baby, the more your confidence will increase. Of course, the community midwife and then the health visitor and your own GP are there to advise you should you have any worries or problems.

COPING

'Everybody tells you how much having a baby's going to disrupt your life, your relationships – especially with your partner – but I didn't find that. Obviously, when you're both tired, nerves get frayed, but life's tons better with a baby than without.'

(A FATHER)

INVOLVING YOUR PARTNER

The more you can share your baby's care, the more you will both enjoy your baby. Your partner may not be able to breastfeed but he can help with bathing, changing and dressing as well as cuddling and playing. He may feel quite nervous of handling the baby and need encouragement. Be patient if he seems awkward at first.

HELP AT HOME

You'll probably need a lot of full-time help at first, not just with the chores, but also to give you emotional support. You're bound to feel up and down and to get easily tired in the early days. Many women

want to have their partners with them so that they will have a chance to get to know the baby properly, as well as helping with the work. It also gives you some time to start adjusting to the changes in your life. If you're on your own, or your partner is unable to be with you, perhaps your mother or a close friend can be there. Even with help you will probably feel tired. Cut corners where you can.

- **Cut down on cleaning.** A bit of dust won't hurt.

- **Keep meals simple.** You need to eat well but this needn't involve a great deal of preparation and cooking.

- **Try to space visitors out.** Too many in a short time will be very tiring. If visitors do come, don't feel you have to tidy up or lay on a meal. Let them do things for you.

- **If you need extra help, ask.** Friends or neighbours will probably be very willing to do some shopping, for example.

LOOKING AFTER YOURSELF

REST

During the weeks or months that you are feeding your baby at night and your body is recovering from childbirth, finding time to catch up on rest is essential. It's tempting to use your baby's sleep times to catch up on chores, but try to have a sleep or a proper rest at least once a day.

PHYSICAL ACTIVITY

Continue with the postnatal exercises you were shown in hospital. You'll begin to benefit quite soon if you keep them up and they shouldn't be difficult to fit in during odd moments. Do your pelvic floor exercises (see page 14) – try doing ten sets of five tightenings a day. You can carry on with the pelvic rocking exercise (see page 14), sitting or standing, but don't kneel. Abdominal exercises to strengthen, firm and flatten your tummy should be done three or four times a day:

- lie on your back, with your feet on the floor, hip–width apart;

- press your back to the floor;

- put both hands on your thighs and curl your head and shoulders off the floor reaching towards your knees;

- breathe out as you go up, and in as you slowly come down;

- do 10 each time to start with, gradually increasing to 20, several times a day.

Besides these exercises, try to fit in a walk with your baby. A short walk in the fresh air will make you feel good.

FOOD

It's very important to continue to eat properly (see pages 8–10). If you want to lose weight, don't rush it. A varied diet without too many fatty foods will help you lose weight gradually. Try to make time to sit down, relax, enjoy your food and digest it properly. It doesn't have to be complicated. Try food like baked potatoes with baked beans and cheese, salads, pasta, french bread pizza, scrambled eggs or sardines on toast, for example, followed by fruit mixed with yoghurt or fromage frais.

A healthy diet is especially important if you're breastfeeding. Breastfeeding uses up a lot of energy. Some of the fat you put on in pregnancy will be used to help produce milk, but the rest of the nutrients will come from your diet. This means that you may be hungrier than usual. If you do need a snack, try having toast with polyunsaturated margarine, cheese on toast, sandwiches, bowls of cereals or fruit.

YOUR RELATIONSHIPS

When you bring your new baby home all the relationships around you will start to shift and change. Your mother, for example, may find the change alarming and feel quite unsure of how much to get involved. You may find that she is trying to take you over or that she is so anxious to avoid bothering you that she doesn't help at all. Try to let the people close to you know clearly just how much you do want from them.

Your relationship with your partner will also change. It's very easy in those exhausting early weeks to just leave things to sort themselves out. Take care. You may wake up six months later to find that you haven't spent an hour alone together and have lost the easy knack of talking your problems through. You both need time alone, without the baby, to recharge your own batteries, and time together to keep in touch with each other.

Your relationship with the baby may not be easy either, particularly if you're not getting much sleep. Don't feel guilty if you sometimes feel resentful at the demands your baby makes, or if your feelings are not what you expected them to be. Talk to your midwife or health visitor if you're upset, but remember, many mothers do not feel instant love for their baby. They come to love them gradually over the weeks.

THE BABY BLUES AND POSTNATAL DEPRESSION

Up to 80% of mothers go through a patch of what is known as the 'baby blues', often about three or four days after the birth. You might feel very anxious about small things, for example, or mildly depressed or just keep bursting into tears, for no apparent reason.

Baby blues may be caused by hormone changes, tiredness, discomfort from sore stitches or sore breasts or even a feeling of anti-climax after all the excitement. Whatever the cause, you will usually find it only lasts a day or so. Have a good cry if you feel like it, and try to sleep if you can. The best help your partner or someone close can give is probably just to listen, give you a reassuring hug and look after the baby while you get some rest. If these feelings do not go away, it may be that you are simply not treating yourself very well. Take time out for treats, however small – a long lazy bath, your favourite food or visit a friend.

Around 10% of mothers slide into a depression which may be quite deep. They are taken over by a feeling of hopelessness. They may feel angry, but more often feel too exhausted to be angry or even to cope with the simplest tasks. If you feel like this you must get help. You, or your partner or friends, should contact your GP or health visitor and explain how you are feeling. You can also contact the Association for Post–Natal Illness (see page 136) for more information.

SEX AND CONTRACEPTION

There are no rules about when to start making love again. If you haven't had stitches you may be eager to share the extra love you feel with your partner. On the other hand, if you're tired and sore, sex may be the last thing you have in mind. Don't rush into it. If it hurts, it will be no pleasure. You may want to use a lubricating jelly the first time because hormone changes may make your vagina feel drier than usual.

It can take some time for the old feelings to come back but they will and, until they do, you may both feel happier finding other ways of being loving and close. If you have any worries, discuss them with your GP or health visitor.

It's possible for a woman to conceive even if she has not started her periods again or even if she is breastfeeding. Contraception should be discussed before you leave hospital and again when you go for your six-week postnatal check. In the meantime, you could talk to your midwife or health visitor when they visit you at home or you could go to your GP or family planning clinic.

The Family Planning Association (see page 136) publishes free leaflets about all methods of contraception.

...but won't the baby wake up?

POSSIBLE METHODS OF CONTRACEPTION

- **The condom** – *this may be the best and simplest choice for the early weeks after childbirth.*

- **The combined pill** – *if you're not breastfeeding, start taking this pill from the 21st day after delivery. If you start it later than the 21st day, it won't be reliable for the first seven days, so for this time you'll have to use some other form of contraceptive (like a condom) as well. Don't take this pill if you're breastfeeding as it reduces the milk flow.*

- **Progestogen-only pill** – *if you're breastfeeding, you may be offered a progestogen-only pill which will not affect your milk supply. This is also started on the 21st day after delivery and has to be taken at the same time every day. There's no evidence to suggest that this pill affects the baby in any way but, even so, some women prefer not to take any form of contraceptive pill while they are breastfeeding and use another form of contraception instead.*

- **Cap or diaphragm** – *these can be used six weeks after delivery. Your old one probably won't fit. Have a new one fitted at your postnatal check-up.*

- **IUD (Intrauterine device)** – *this can be fitted at your postnatal check-up when the womb is back to its normal size.*

113

THE POSTNATAL VISIT

You should have your postnatal visit about six weeks after your baby's birth to make sure that you feel well and are recovering as you should from the birth. You may go to your own GP or may be asked to return to the hospital. It's a good opportunity to ask any questions and sort out any problems that are troubling you. You may like to make a list of questions to take along with you so that you don't forget what you want to ask.

Routines do vary a little but the list below is probably what will be done.

- You may be **weighed**. You may be on the way to getting back to your normal weight again by now. Breastfeeding mothers tend to lose weight more quickly than those who are bottle feeding.

- Your **urine** may be tested to make sure your kidneys are working properly and that there is no infection.

- Your **blood pressure** will be checked.

- You may be offered an examination to see whether your **stitches** (if you had any) have healed, whether your **womb** is back to its normal size, and whether all the **muscles** used during labour and delivery are returning to normal. Tell the doctor if the examination is uncomfortable.

- Your **breasts** may be examined.

- The **cervical smear test** may be discussed if you haven't had one in the past three years (see page 51). This is usually delayed until three months after delivery.

- If you are not **immune to rubella** (German measles) and were not given an immunisation before you left hospital, you will be offered one now. You should not become pregnant for one month after this immunisation.

- The doctor will ask if you still have any **vaginal discharge** and whether you have had a **period** yet.

- There will be an opportunity to talk about **contraception**. If you have any worries over contraception or, indeed, any aspect of sex, now is a good time to discuss them.

- If you're feeling **very tired, low or depressed** make sure you tell the doctor about this.

Babies are quite often brought along to postnatal clinics, so don't worry if you can't find a babysitter. Your GP would probably like to see your baby anyway.

16 The early weeks: your baby

The baby's birth must be registered within six weeks from the date of birth at your nearest Registry Office. The address will be in the telephone book under the name of your local authority (in Northern Ireland, look under 'Registration of births, deaths and marriages'). If you are married, you or the father can register the birth. If you are not married you must go yourself, and if you want the father's name to appear on the birth certificate he must go with you.

REGISTERING THE BIRTH

If you live in a different district from the one where your baby was born, the registrar will take details from you and then send them to the district where the birth took place. You will then be sent the birth certificate. You cannot claim benefits or register your baby with a doctor until you have a birth certificate and a National Health Service number which will be issued at the same time. In Scotland a birth must be registered within three weeks. This can either be in the district where the baby was born or in the district where the parents live.

CRYING

All babies cry. It's their way of saying that something isn't right. Sometimes you'll be able to find the reason for your baby's distress and deal with it. At other times all you can do is try to comfort or distract your baby. If it's not obvious why your baby is crying, think of possible reasons. Could it be:

- hunger?
- wet or dirty nappy?
- wind?
- colic?
- feeling hot, cold or uncomfortable?
- feeling tired and unable to sleep?
- feeling lonely and wanting company?
- feeling bored and wanting to play?

'I think there must be something there even before the birth. But it builds up as well. You know, it takes time to form a bond and over the months and years it grows stronger.'

115

'I think it has changed me. I think I've got a wider outlook on life now than I did before. And I can speak more openly to people. I can speak more freely. I'm more patient, too, whereas before I was very quick-tempered.'

It could be none of these things. Perhaps your baby simply feels overwhelmed and a bit frightened by all the new sights, sounds and sensations in the early weeks of life and needs time to adjust. Holding your baby close and talking in a soothing voice or singing softly will be reassuring.

Movement often helps to calm down crying. Gently sway or rock your baby or take your baby for a walk in the pram or baby carrier or even for a ride in a car. Sucking can

also be comforting. You can put your baby to your breast or give your baby a dummy if you wish. But if you do, make sure it is sterilised.

Do not dip the dummy in honey or sugar to make your baby suck – he or she will suck anyway. Using sugar will only encourage a craving for sweet things which are harmful to children's teeth.

Some babies do cry more than others and it's not really clear why. Don't blame yourself or your baby if he or she cries a lot. It can be very exhausting so try to get rest when

you can. Share soothing your baby with your partner. You could ask a friend or relative to take over for an hour from time to time, just to give you a break. If there's no one to turn to and you feel your patience is running out, leave your baby in the cot, put on some music to drown the noise, and go into another room for a few minutes. Make yourself a cup of tea, telephone a friend or find some other way to unwind. You'll cope better if you do.

Never shake your baby. Shaking makes a baby's head move violently. It can cause bleeding and damage the brain. Put the baby down safely in a cot or pram and calm yourself; don't be angry with the baby. If you feel you're having difficulties in coping with your baby's crying, talk to your midwife or health visitor. Or contact CRY–SIS (see page 136) who will put you in touch with other parents who've been in the same situation.

If your baby's crying sounds different or unusual, it may be the first sign of illness, particularly if the baby isn't feeding well or won't be comforted. If you think your baby is ill, contact your doctor immediately. In an emergency, if you cannot contact your doctor, take your baby to the nearest hospital Accident and Emergency Department.

SLEEPING

The amount babies sleep, even when they are very small, varies a lot. During the early weeks some babies sleep for most of the time between feeds. Others will be wide awake. As they grow older they begin to develop a pattern of waking and sleeping which changes as time goes by. Some babies need more sleep than others and at different times.

You'll gradually begin to recognise when your baby is ready for sleep and is likely to settle. Some babies settle better after a warm bath. Most sleep after a good feed. A baby who wants to sleep isn't likely to be disturbed by ordinary household noises, so there's no need to keep your whole home quiet while your baby sleeps. It will help you if your baby can get used to sleeping through a certain amount of noise.

See below for advice on sleeping positions.

REDUCING THE RISK OF COT DEATH

Sadly, we don't yet know why some babies die suddenly and for no apparent reason from what is called cot death or Sudden Infant Death Syndrome (SIDS). This section lists, in detail, all the advice we now have for reducing the risk of cot death as well as other dangers such as suffocation. There are three ways in which you can reduce the risk:

- **always put babies to sleep on their backs**

- **avoid dressing your baby too warmly or overheating the room**

- **do not smoke or allow others to smoke near your baby or the room your baby sleeps in.**

A SAFE PLACE TO SLEEP

Babies should always be put to sleep on their *backs* unless there is clear medical advice to do something different. Babies sleeping on their backs are *not* more likely to choke, and the risk of cot death is greatly increased for babies sleeping on

their fronts. Keep your baby's head uncovered and place your baby in the 'feet to foot' position to prevent your baby wriggling under the covers. Make the cot so that the covers reach no higher than your baby's shoulders.

The 'feet to foot' position means that the baby's feet are right at the end of the cot to prevent the baby wriggling under the covers.

Ask your doctor or midwife for the leaflet, *Reduce the risk of cot death*, published by the Department of Health and FSID.

THE RIGHT TEMPERATURE

Small babies are not very good at controlling their own temperature. It's just as important to avoid getting too hot as it is to avoid getting chilled. Overheating is known to be a factor in cot death. Remember:

- if the room is warm enough for you to be comfortable wearing light clothing (16–20°C) then it is the right temperature for your baby;

- give your baby one light layer of clothing (or bedding) more than you are wearing. If the room is too hot for you, keep your baby's clothes or bed-covering light;

- don't use duvets (quilts) until your baby is a year old – they get too hot;

- keep your baby's head uncovered (unless it's very cold) as babies need to lose heat from their heads and faces;

- never use a hot water bottle or electric blanket as babies have delicate skin which can scald easily;

- ill or feverish babies do *not* need any extra bedding – in fact, they usually need less;

- there has been some advice suggesting that it is unwise to have your baby in bed with you – there is no clear evidence of risk, but it would be wise not to have your baby in your bed if you have been drinking alcohol or have taken drugs which can cause drowsiness, and to be careful not to get the baby too hot;

- babies chill easily if it's cold, so wrap them up well when you go out, but **remember to take off the extra clothing when you come back inside**, even if you have to wake your baby to do it;

- avoid plastic sheets or bumpers, ribbons and bits of string from mobiles anywhere near your baby, who could get entangled in them;

- make sure there's no gap between the cot mattress and the sides of the cot which your baby's body could slip through;

- remove any loose plastic covering from the mattress which could come off and smother your baby.

You can protect your children by keeping their playing, sleeping and eating areas completely smoke free.

CLEAN AIR

Babies should not be exposed to tobacco smoke, either before birth or afterwards. If you, or anyone else who looks after your baby, smoke then don't smoke anywhere near the baby. Ask friends to smoke outside or before visiting you. It would be even better if everyone could make an effort to give up completely.

Babies and young children who breathe in cigarette smoke are also more likely to get coughs, asthma and chest infections. For more advice on giving up smoking, see page 11.

COT MATTRESSES

There have been suggestions that toxic gases from fire-retardant materials found in some cot mattresses are another potential cause of cot death. These suggestions are currently being examined. However, recent studies have not found any evidence that using PVC mattresses causes cot death.

Following the advice given above will help to reduce the risk of cot death.

If your baby seems at all unwell, seek medical advice early and quickly.

Do remember that cot death is rare. Don't let worrying about cot death spoil the first precious months you have with your baby.

NAPPIES

Babies need their nappies changed fairly often, otherwise they become sore. Unless your baby is sleeping peacefully, always change a wet or dirty nappy and change your baby before or after each feed, whichever you prefer.

Organise the place where you change your baby so that everything you need is handy (see page 81). If you're using terry nappies, your midwife or your friends can show you different ways of folding them. Experiment to find out which method is easiest and best for you.

CHANGING NAPPIES

You need to clean your baby's bottom carefully each time you change a nappy to help prevent soreness.

- Take off the nappy. If it's dirty, wipe away the mess from your baby's bottom with tissues or cotton wool.

- Wash your baby's bottom and genitals with cotton wool and warm water and dry thoroughly. Or use baby lotion. For girls, wipe the bottom from front to back, away from the vagina so that germs won't infect the vagina or bladder. For boys, gently clean the foreskin of the penis, but don't pull it back; clean under the penis and the scrotum.

- You may want to use a cream such as zinc and castor oil cream which forms a waterproof coating to help protect the skin. Or you can just leave the skin clean and dry.

- Don't use baby powder as it can cause choking.

- If you're using a terry nappy, fold it and put a nappy liner inside, if you wish. Pin the corners of the nappy together with a proper nappy pin which won't spring open.

- If you use disposable nappies, be very careful not to get cream on the tabs or they won't stick down.

- Put on, or tie on, the plastic pants, if you're using a terry nappy.

- Wash your hands.

NAPPY HYGIENE

Disposable nappies
If the nappy is dirty, flush the contents down the toilet. Roll up the nappy and re-tape it securely. Put it into a plastic bag kept only for this purpose. Fasten the bag and put it outside in your bin each day.

Terry nappies
- If the nappy is dirty, flush the contents down the toilet and rinse off the nappy in the flushing water.

- Have a plastic bucket (with a lid) ready filled with water and the right amount of nappy sanitising powder. Follow the instructions on the packet. Make sure you keep the nappy powder out of reach of small children.

- Put the dirty nappy to soak in the bucket.

- Wash each day's nappies in very hot water. Don't use enzyme (bio) washing powders as these may irritate your baby's skin. Rinse very thoroughly. Don't use fabric conditioners as they may also irritate the skin.

NAPPY RASH

Most babies get soreness or a nappy rash at some time, but some have extra sensitive skins. If you notice redness or spots, clean your baby very carefully and change nappies more frequently. Better still, give your baby time without a nappy and let the air get to the skin (keep a spare nappy handy to mop up). You will soon see the rash start to get better.

If your baby does have a rash, ask your midwife or health visitor about it. They may advise you to use a protective cream. If the rash seems to be painful and won't go away, see your GP.

PUTTING ON A DISPOSABLE NAPPY

With disposables, the end with the sticky tapes goes under your baby's bottom. Fasten the tapes at the front.

PUTTING ON A TERRY NAPPY

Lay your baby carefully on to a clean nappy and liner.

Bring the centre of the nappy between your baby's legs and then bring over the first side piece.

Bring over the second side piece and fasten all three pieces together with a nappy pin. Put on plastic pants over the top.

BABIES' STOOLS

You can't really explain, but it's a most wonderful thing to be a mum. To look after a baby and rear her, watching the different little things she does every day. It's just fantastic.'

Immediately after birth, and for the first few days, your baby is likely to pass a sticky black-green substance. This is called meconium and it is the waste that has collected in the bowels during the time spent in the womb.

As your baby begins to digest milk, the stools will change, probably becoming more yellow or orange. The colours can be quite bright. Breastfed babies have quite runny stools. Bottle–fed babies' stools are firmer and smell more.

Babies vary a lot in how often they pass stools. Some have a bowel movement at or around each feed; some can go for several days without having a movement. Either can be normal.

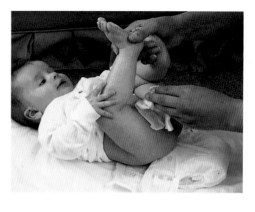

Most small babies strain and go red in the face, or even cry, when passing a stool. This is normal and doesn't mean they are constipated so long as the stools are soft. If you are worried that your baby may be constipated, mention this to your midwife or health visitor.

What you find in your baby's nappies will probably vary from day to day and usually there is no need to worry about how runny the stools are, for example. But if you notice a marked change of any kind in your baby's bowel movements, such as the stools becoming very frequent and watery or particularly smelly or if they change colour to become green, white or creamy, for example, then you should get advice from your doctor, midwife or health visitor. (See page 109, **Babies with jaundice after two weeks**.)

Is it really supposed to look like that?

WASHING AND BATHING

WASHING

You don't need to bath your baby every day but you should wash your baby's face, neck, hands and bottom carefully each day. You can do this on your lap or on a changing mat. Choose a time when your baby is awake and contented and make sure the room is warm. You'll need a bowl of warm water, some cotton wool, a towel and a fresh nappy.

1 Take off your baby's clothes except for the vest and nappy. Wrap the baby in a towel.

2 Gently wipe round each eye, from the nose side outwards, using a fresh piece of cotton wool for each eye.

3 Using fresh, moist cotton wool again, wipe out each ear but don't clean inside the ears.

4 Wash the rest of your baby's face and neck with moist cotton wool and gently dry. Wash and dry your baby's hands in the same way.

5 Take off the nappy and wash your baby's genitals, again with cotton wool and warm water. Dry very carefully and put on a fresh nappy. In the first week or so, you should also clean round the navel each day. Your midwife will show you how.

BATHING

Bath your baby two or three times a week, or more often if your baby enjoys it. Don't bath straight after a feed or when your baby is hungry or sleepy. Make sure the room is warm and that you have everything you need ready in advance.

- Check that the water is not too hot, just comfortably warm to your wrist or elbow.

- Undress your baby, except for a nappy, and wrap snugly in a towel. Wash your baby's face with cotton wool and water as described above. Don't use soap on your baby's face.

- Wash your baby's hair with baby soap or liquid, supporting the head over the baby bath or basin. Rinse carefully.

- If you're using baby soap, unwrap your baby and soap all over, still on your lap so you have a firm grip. Take the nappy off at the last minute. If you're using baby bath liquid add it to the water at this stage.

- Put your baby gently into the water. Using one hand for support, gently swish the water to wash your baby without splashing the face. You should *never* leave your baby alone in the water even for a few seconds.

- Lift your baby out and pat dry with the towel. Dry carefully in all the creases. If your baby's skin is dry, gently massage in some baby oil. Your baby may enjoy this anyway.

- **Never leave your baby alone in the bath.**

If your baby seems frightened of the bath and cries, it may help to try bathing together. You may like to do this anyway. Make sure the water is only warm, not hot, and don't add anything to the water unless it's baby bath liquid.

ILLNESS

It's sometimes difficult to tell at first when a baby is ill but you may have a funny feeling that things aren't quite right. If you're at all worried, ask for help. You are not fussing. It's far better to be on the safe side, particularly with a very small baby. Trust your own judgement. You know your baby best.

VERY URGENT PROBLEMS

Sometimes there are more obvious signs that your baby is not well. Contact your doctor at once if your baby:

- makes jerky movements – this is a fit or convulsion;

- turns blue or very pale;

- has quick, difficult or grunting breathing, or unusual periods of breathing, for example if your baby breathes with pauses of over 20 seconds between breaths;

- is very hard to wake, or unusually drowsy, or doesn't seem to know you;

- develops a rash of red spots which do not fade and lose colour (blanch) when they are pressed. This may be the rash of meningococcal septicaemia – an infection in the blood.

There may not be any other symptoms (see photo). Your baby may need treatment very quickly. If you can't get hold of your GP at once, dial 999 for an ambulance or take your baby to the Accident and Emergency Department of your nearest hospital as quickly as possible.

PROBLEMS THAT COULD BE SERIOUS

- If your baby has a hoarse cough with noisy breathing, is wheezing, or cannot breathe through the nose.

- If your baby is unusually hot, cold or floppy.

- If your baby cries in an unusual way or for an unusually long time or seems to be in pain.

- If you notice any bleeding from the stump of the cord or from the nose, or any bruising.

- If your baby keeps refusing feeds.

- If your baby keeps vomiting a substantial part of feeds or has frequent watery diarrhoea. Vomiting and diarrhoea together may mean your baby is losing too much fluid and this may need prompt treatment.

- If your baby develops jaundice (looks yellow) when it is over a week old.

If you have seen your GP and your baby is not getting better or seems to be getting worse, tell your GP again the same day. If you become very worried and can't get hold of your GP or your GP can't get to you quickly enough, dial 999 for an ambulance or take your baby to the Accident and Emergency

WHERE TO GET SUPPORT

Department of the nearest hospital. Everyone needs advice or reassurance at some time or other when they are caring for a young baby, even if it's just to make sure that they are doing the right thing. Some problems just need talking over with someone. It's always better to ask for help than worry on your own. Do talk to your midwife or health visitor. As you grow more confident, you'll begin to trust your own judgement more. You will be able to decide which advice makes most sense for you and your baby and which suggestions you can safely ignore.

You will also want to talk to friends, relations or other mothers in a similar situation. You'll meet other mothers when you start taking your baby to the Child Health Clinic. Your health visitor will explain where this is and when you should go. The health visitor can also tell you about any mother and baby groups in the area. Or your local branch of the National Childbirth Trust (see page 134) or MAMA (Meet-A-Mum Association) (see page 135) may be able to put you in touch with other mothers nearby.

SUNSHINE

In warm, sunny weather, always protect your baby from direct sunlight with a sunhat or sunshade. Never leave your baby in a place where he or she could become overheated.

Remember too that a baby's skin burns easily, even in sun that would not affect your own. Consider using a high protection sunblock (sun protection factor 15+) to help protect your baby's skin from the sun.

ENJOYING YOUR BABY

So far we have only talked about the things that have to be done to keep your baby warm, fed and safe. In the first weeks those things can grow to fill all the available time, but of course they're only a tiny part of what it means to be a parent. Every second that your baby is awake he or she is learning from you. Learning about what it feels like to be touched gently, about the sound of your voice and your very special smell, about what the world is like and whether it is a safe place to be and, above all, what it feels like to love and be loved.

123

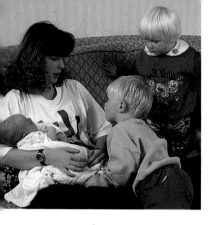

17 Thinking about the next baby?

DIFFICULTY CONCEIVING

It can take several months or more to conceive even if it happened really quickly the first time.

If you're feeling very tired looking after the first baby, it may be that you are simply not making love at the right time. Re-read the section on Conception (pages 18-22) to remind yourself when you are most likely to succeed. If nothing happens after a few months, and you feel anxious about it, talk to your doctor or family planning clinic.

As you hold your new baby in your arms, it may be impossible to imagine that you will ever have the energy to go through it all again. Or you may be eager to increase your family as soon as you can. Either way, this is the time to stop and think about how you and your partner can prepare for the next pregnancy. Nobody can guarantee that a baby will be born healthy. However, if you had a low birthweight baby or a baby with a disability or special needs, or a miscarriage or stillbirth, you may be particularly anxious to do everything you can to create the best possible circumstances for your next pregnancy. You'll want to talk to your doctor about this. If both parents are in good health at the moment of conception, that is the best start you can possibly give to a new life. There are a few other steps you can take as well.

FATHERS TOO

A bad diet, smoking, drinking and unhealthy working conditions can affect the quality of sperm and stop pregnancy from happening at all. Try to make your lifestyle as healthy as possible before you try to conceive.

GETTING AND STAYING HEALTHY

Re-read Chapter 1, **Your health in pregnancy,** about diet, smoking, alcohol and exercise. The advice is even more effective if you start well before the next baby is on the way. You will need to prepare for pregnancy by taking extra folic acid from the time you start trying to conceive right up until you're 12 weeks pregnant. Choose foods that

124

contain this important vitamin such as green, leafy vegetables and breakfast cereals and breads with added folic acid. To make sure you get enough, you should also take a 400 microgram (0.4 milligram) tablet every day. You can get these tablets from a pharmacist. If you already have a baby with spina bifida, if you have coeliac disease or take anti-epileptic drugs, ask your GP for more advice, since you will need to take a bigger dose of folic acid.

THINGS TO THINK ABOUT

Here are some things that are worth doing before having your next baby.

Rubella (German measles)
Rubella can badly damage a baby during pregnancy. If you were not already immune you should have been offered immunisation immediately after your baby was born. Before trying for another baby, think about having a blood test to check that you are immune to rubella. The blood test will measure if you have enough protection (antibodies) against rubella. Women with low or uncertain levels of antibodies can be immunised again.

Long-term medication
If either of you has a chronic illness or disability and has to take long-term medication, talk to your doctor in advance of pregnancy about any possible effects on fertility or pregnancy. It may be possible to cut down the dosage.

Diabetes and epilepsy
If you have diabetes or epilepsy, talk to your doctor in advance.

Medicines and drugs
These may endanger your baby's health. Don't take any over-the-counter drugs at the time you hope to conceive without making sure that they are safe to take in pregnancy. Addictive drugs will affect your ability to conceive and, if you do conceive, are likely to damage your baby's health. See page 136 for organisations which can help you to stop.

Sexually transmitted infections (STIs)
STIs can affect your ability to conceive as well as affecting you. If there is any chance that either of you has been in contact with an STI, it's important to get it diagnosed and treated before starting another pregnancy. STIs, including HIV and hepatitis B, can be passed on through:

- sexual intercourse with an infected person, especially without using a condom. Some STIs can be transmitted during sex without penetration;
- HIV and hepatitis B can also be passed on by sharing injected drugs equipment.

If you're HIV positive, you could pass the virus on to your baby either in the womb, at birth, or by breastfeeding. About 15% of children born to mothers with the virus are likely to be infected (see box, page 50).

HAZARDS AT WORK

If you or your partner think there may be a risk involved in your work, talk to a union representative, your employer or personnel department. You have a legal right to know whether there is a definite risk. If there is a risk, ask if you can be moved to a safer job or, if this is not possible, find out whether wearing protective clothing, avoiding breathing in fumes and dust, and avoiding skin contact provide sufficient protection.

18 Rights and benefits

I t's very important that you get help and advice as soon as you know that you're pregnant, to make sure that you claim all the benefits to which you are entitled. Benefits have to be claimed on a lot of different forms, from a lot of different offices, and the situation is always changing. The figures given here are accurate up to March 1998.

There are many voluntary organisations that are happy to help. Don't hesitate to ask for advice. If in doubt, get a second opinion. See the box below on where to get advice.

BENEFITS FOR ALL

WHERE TO GET ADVICE AND HELP

Working out what benefits you are entitled to and making claims can be complicated. Get help if you need it.

- *You can go to your local social security office (look in the phone book under 'Benefits Agency'; in Northern Ireland 'Social Security Agency'). Or go to your local Citizens' Advice Bureau or other advice centre (see page 134). Social security offices can be very busy and an advice centre is often the best place to go.*

- *Some local authorities have welfare officers. Phone your social services department (in Scotland social work department, in Northern Ireland local Health and Social Services Board) and ask.*

- *Some voluntary organisations offer information and advice on benefits. For example, the National Council for One Parent Families, the Scottish Council for Single Parents and the Maternity Alliance (see page 134).*

Prescriptions and NHS dental treatment are free during pregnancy, for a year after the birth, and for all children. To claim for prescriptions, ask your GP or midwife for form FW8 and send it to your Health Authority (in Scotland, Health Board; in Northern Ireland, Central Services Agency). To claim for dental treatment, simply tell your dentist that you are pregnant or have a child under one year old.

CHILD BENEFIT

What is it?
A tax-free benefit paid weekly for each child. It is payable from birth.

Who gets it?
Every mother.

How much is it?
£11.05 a week for your first child if you are in a couple, or £17.10 a week for your first child if you are a lone parent (not living with someone as husband and wife). For other children you get £9.00 a week per child.

How do I claim?
You may receive a Child Benefit claim pack automatically. If you do not, then you can get one from your social security office or post office. Or you can use the form on the back of the leaflet *Babies and benefits* which you can get from post offices and clinics. You need to send your baby's birth certificate (see page 115). It will be returned to you.

IF YOUR INCOME IS LOW

INCOME-BASED JOBSEEKER'S ALLOWANCE ('JSA') AND INCOME SUPPORT ('IS')

What are they?
Weekly payments for people who do not have enough money to live on.

Who gets them?
You can claim JSA if you are over 18, *and* unemployed or working for less than 16 hours a week, *and* you are actively seeking work. If you are 16 or 17 years old you can claim JSA once your baby is born (but if you're single it's better to claim IS), or earlier if you face severe hardship.

You can claim IS if you are over 16, *and* you're a lone parent, *or* you're pregnant and incapable of work, *or* you're pregnant and within the period of 11 weeks before the baby is due until 7 weeks after the baby is born. You do not have to be available for work.

You cannot claim Income-based JSA or IS if you have a partner who works for more than 24 hours a week or if you have savings of more than £8,000.

How much is it?
It depends on your age and the size of your family. If you're under 25 you get a lower rate. The amount will be reduced if you have savings over £3,000. If you're earning or claiming other benefits such as Statutory Maternity Pay or Maternity Allowance, your income will be 'topped up' to the JSA/IS level for your family size.

How do I claim?
Claim JSA by going to the JobCentre in person (postal applications are allowed if you live too far from the JobCentre). In Northern Ireland claim JSA at your local social security office. Claim IS on form A1 which you can get from a social security office or post office. Return it to your social security office.

FAMILY CREDIT

What is it?
A tax-free benefit for working families on low pay who have children.

Who gets it?
Families (including one-parent families) with at least one child where one parent works 16 hours a week or more.

How much is it?
It depends on the size of your family, your income and your savings. A couple with one baby may get Family Credit if their earnings (after tax) are less than about £160 a week. If you or your partner work 30 hours or more per week you may get Family Credit if your family income is less than £175 per week. If you pay for a registered childminder to look after your child, you may be able to earn up to £60 more and still get Family Credit. The more children you have and the older they get, the more you can earn and still get Family Credit. You cannot get Family Credit if you have savings of over £8,000 and you get less if you have savings of over £3,000.

How do I claim?
Claim on form FC1 which you can get from post offices and social security offices. Post the form in the envelope provided.

If you get Income-based Jobseeker's Allowance, Income Support, or Family Credit, or have a low income, you may also be able to get other benefits:

A MATERNITY PAYMENT

What is it?
This is a one-off payment from the Social Fund to help you buy things for your baby. You can claim from 11 weeks before the birth to three months afterwards. If you can't get Income-based Jobseeker's Allowance, Income Support or Family Credit until after your baby is born, claim the Maternity Payment within three months after the birth.

How much is it?
£100. You get less if you have savings of over £500. For every £1 of savings over £500, £1 will be deducted.

How do I claim?
Claim on form SF100 which you can get from social security offices. Send your maternity certificate, MAT B1, which you get from your GP or midwife when you're about six months pregnant. If you're claiming after the birth, send the baby's birth certificate. It will be returned to you.

HOUSING BENEFIT

What is it?
Housing Benefit will help you pay your rent (and/or rates in Northern Ireland) if you're on Income-based Jobseeker's Allowance, Income Support, Family Credit or a low income. It will be paid direct to the council if you're a council tenant, or in Northern Ireland to the Northern Ireland Housing Executive if you're a Housing

Executive tenant, or to you or your landlord if you're a private tenant.

If you've got a mortgage and you're on Income-based Jobseeker's Allowance or Income Support, you may be able to get help with your mortgage interest payments. See leaflet IS8 *Help with housing costs* (available from your social security office) for details.

How much is it?
It depends on your income, savings, other benefits and family size. It may not be the same amount as the rent you are actually paying.

How do I claim?
If you're getting Jobseeker's Allowance or Income Support you will get a Housing Benefit claim form with your JSA/IS claim form. Otherwise get a form from your local council. In Northern Ireland if you're not claiming JSA/IS get an HB1 form from your Northern Ireland Housing Executive district office (for tenants) or the Rate Collection Agency, Londonderry House, 21-27 Chichester Street, Belfast BT1 4UX (if you own your own home).

COUNCIL TAX BENEFIT
(Not applicable in Northern Ireland)

What is it?
A benefit to help you pay your Council Tax.

Who gets it?
If your income is low or you're getting Family Credit, Income-based Jobseeker's Allowance or Income Support, you could get Council Tax Benefit.

How much is it?
You may get all of your Council Tax paid or just part of it. It will depend on your income, savings, whether other adults live with you, and an assessment of your circumstances.

How do I claim?
If you're getting Jobseeker's Allowance or Income Support you will get a Council Tax claim form with your JSA/IS claim form. Otherwise get a form from your local council.

FREE MILK AND VITAMINS

What is it and who gets it?
If you're on Income-based Jobseeker's Allowance or Income Support, you can get tokens for one free pint of milk a day for yourself while you are pregnant or breastfeeding, and for each child under the age

of five. If you want normal milk you can exchange the tokens at any shop or milkman who will take them. If your baby is under one year old and you are bottle feeding, you can exchange the tokens for dried baby milk at a maternity or child health clinic, a welfare food distribution centre or some pharmacies.

How do I claim?
If you or someone in your family becomes pregnant, you should tell the social security office and let them know the date the baby is due. Show them proof from the doctor or midwife. If you collect your benefit from the post office you can collect your milk tokens at the same time, or they will be posted to you if your benefit is paid directly into your bank account.

You can also get free vitamins for yourself while you're pregnant or breastfeeding, and for any children under the age of five. Vitamin supplements should only be taken on the advice of your GP, midwife or health visitor. You get them from a maternity or child health clinic, from a welfare food distribution centre or from some pharmacies. You do not need tokens but you may need to show proof that you are entitled (your benefit book or

notice of award of benefit) and proof of your children's ages (such as the birth certificate or child benefit order book).

Cheap dried baby milk
If you're getting Family Credit and you've got a child under one year old who you're bottle feeding, you can buy dried baby milk at a reduced price. Take your Family Credit order book or notice of award to your local maternity or child health clinic, or welfare food distribution centre or some pharmacies to prove that you're getting Family Credit. You may also have to prove your baby's age for example by showing the birth certificate or child benefit order book. For further information see leaflet WMV:GI *Free milk and vitamins: a guide for families* (in Northern Ireland leaflet WMV:GI (NI).

HELP WITH HOSPITAL FARES

Families on Income-based Jobseeker's Allowance, Income Support, Family Credit or on a low income can get help with fares to and from the antenatal clinic or hospital. See leaflet HC11 *Are you entitled to help with NHS costs?* which you can get from your social security office or hospital.

EMPLOYMENT RIGHTS AND BENEFITS

As a working mother-to-be, you are entitled to maternity leave, protection against unfair dismissal for pregnancy-related reasons, and protection against any risks to your health and safety in the workplace. You may also be entitled to claim maternity pay when you stop work to have your baby.

The information in this section tells you what rights and benefits you can claim and how to go about it. Your union representative, employer or personnel department will be able to tell you if your workplace maternity rights are better than the legal minimum. You have the same rights to maternity leave and pay if your baby is stillborn after the 24th week of pregnancy.

14 WEEKS MATERNITY LEAVE

Who gets it?
Every woman who is employed while she is pregnant is entitled to 14 weeks maternity leave. When you return to work you will go back to the same job. This right applies to every employee who gives the required notice (see below). You don't need to work a certain number of hours a week, or to have worked for the same employer for a specified length of time in order to qualify.

How do I get it?
Write to your employer *at least* 21 days before you start your maternity leave telling them
(1) that you are pregnant and
(2) giving them the expected date of childbirth.
You must also tell them
(3) the date you intend to start your maternity leave (you only need to put this in writing if your employer asks for it).
Finally you must, if your employer asks for it
(4) enclose a copy of your maternity certificate (form MAT B1) which your midwife or GP will give to you when you are about six months pregnant.
If you cannot give 21 days' notice, for example if you have to go into hospital unexpectedly, you must write to your employer as soon as you reasonably can.

HAVING TIME OFF FOR ANTENATAL CARE

All pregnant women (whatever hours they work and however recently they started the job) have the right to take time off work to attend antenatal appointments, without losing any pay. This includes relaxation classes and parentcraft classes and the time needed to travel to your clinic or GP. Your employer may want to see a letter from your GP, midwife or health visitor, saying that these classes are part of your antenatal care.

You should let your employer know when you need time off and how long you are likely to be away. After your first appointment, your employer can ask to see your appointment card and a certificate signed by your GP, midwife or health visitor, stating that you are pregnant.

If you are not paid or are refused time off you can make a claim to the industrial tribunal within three months.

When can I start it?
The earliest you can start your maternity leave is 11 weeks before the week your baby is due. It's up to you to decide when you want to stop work. You can work right up until the day of childbirth. The only exception to this rule is if you have a pregnancy-related illness absence in the last six weeks of your pregnancy. If this happens you may be bounced on to your maternity leave even if you are away from work for one day. However, if you are ill for only a short time, your employer may agree to let you start your maternity leave on the date you had originally planned.

What will I receive while I'm on leave?
During the 14 weeks maternity leave you will receive all your contractual rights as if you were still at work. This includes holiday entitlement, pension rights and your company car, but you won't receive your normal pay. See pages 132–33 for details of maternity pay.

Returning to work
You don't need to give any notice of your return to work if you are going back at the end of your 14 weeks maternity leave.

If you want to return *before* the end of the 14 weeks you must give your employer seven

1. In this box, write in the date of the Sunday before the first day of your last period. (If your last period started on a Sunday, write in that date.) Then work along the top row filling in the dates of each successive Sunday.

THE TIMING OF YOUR RIGHTS AND BENEFITS IN PREGNANCY IS VERY COMPLICATED, SO USE THIS CHART AS A ROUGH GUIDE ONLY

2. Write in the first day of your last period here. Then work along the row filling in the remaining boxes. Each box represents a week. Write in the dates week by week until you get to the date your baby is due.

days' notice in writing of the date you will be returning. If you don't give this notice and just turn up at work before the end of the 14 weeks, your employer can send you away for seven days or until the end of the 14 weeks, whichever is earlier.

By law, you are not allowed to work for two weeks after giving birth so, if your baby is born very late and your 14 weeks maternity leave runs out, it will be extended by two weeks from the date of the birth of your baby.

If you are sick at the end of your 14 weeks maternity leave and unable to return to work, you can remain off work for up to 4 weeks longer and still be protected from being unfairly dismissed if you have given your employer a sickness certificate. If you are receiving Statutory Maternity Pay (see page 132) you will

continue to receive it for these 4 weeks. If your employer has an occupational sick pay scheme you should get sick pay for these weeks.

EXTENDED MATERNITY ABSENCE

(Up to 29 weeks from the week of childbirth)
You may qualify for more time off work after your baby is born.

Who gets it?
Women who have worked for the same employer for two years by the end of the 12th week before the baby is due, and who carry on working at least until the end of the 12th week. However, women who work in a firm which employs five or fewer people do not have a clear right to return after 29 weeks but they will qualify for 14 weeks maternity leave (see page 129).

How do I get it?
As well as giving notice for your basic 14 weeks maternity leave (see (1)–(4) on page 129), you must also

(5)   tell your employer that you intend to return to work after the birth. (NB this does not mean that you have to return – you can change your mind later). You must put this in writing at least 21 days before you start your leave, but you do not have to give a date for your return at this stage.

How does it work?
The earliest you can leave work is 11 weeks before the expected week of childbirth. You have to return to work by the end of the 29th week from the actual week of childbirth. (Remember to count 29 weeks from the Sunday at the beginning of the

week in which your baby is born.)

Returning to work
Your employer may write to you any time from 11 weeks after the start of your maternity leave asking you to confirm that you are going back to work. You must reply in writing *within* 14 days clearly saying that you are going back, otherwise you will lose that right. (You can still change your mind later).

At least 21 days before you intend to return to work you must write to your employer giving notice of the exact date of your return. This is called your Notified Date of Return. When you return to work your employer must give you back the same job, or if that is not reasonably practicable, a suitable job on similar terms and conditions.

You can only delay your return beyond 29

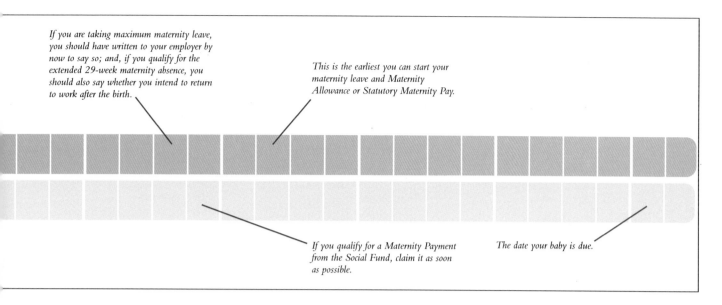

If you are taking maximum maternity leave, you should have written to your employer by now to say so; and, if you qualify for the extended 29-week maternity absence, you should also say whether you intend to return to work after the birth.

This is the earliest you can start your maternity leave and Maternity Allowance or Statutory Maternity Pay.

If you qualify for a Maternity Payment from the Social Fund, claim it as soon as possible.

The date your baby is due.

weeks after the birth in the following circumstances:

- If you are ill you can delay going back for up to four weeks. You must let your employer know before the date on which you had intended to return, that you will be extending your leave because of sickness, and you must send in a medical certificate.

- Your employer can delay your return for up to four weeks. They must tell you the reason for the delay and give you a new date for your return.

- An interruption of work, such as a strike, which stops you returning to work allows you to delay your return until work starts again. If the interruption stops

you giving notice of the date you intend to return, you can delay your return for up to 28 days after the end of the interruption.

- By agreement with your employer.

If you decide not to return to work you should resign and give the normal contractual notice if you can.

DISMISSAL OR UNFAIR TREATMENT

It is against the law for your employer to dismiss you or select you for redundancy for any reason connected with pregnancy, childbirth or maternity leave. It does not matter how long you have worked for your employer or how many hours a week you work.

If you are dismissed while you are pregnant

or during your maternity leave :

- your employer must give you a written statement of the reasons. You should not have to ask for this;

- if you believe the reason is related to your pregnancy, get advice from your trade union or local advice centre. You must put in your claim to the industrial tribunal within three months of dismissal.

If you are sacked or are treated unfairly (for example having your pay cut) because you are pregnant or have had a baby, you may have a claim for sex discrimination. It does not matter how long you have worked for your employer. The law is complicated, so get advice. These claims also have to be made within three months.

HEALTH AND SAFETY RIGHTS FOR PREGNANT WOMEN

If you are pregnant, have given birth within the last six months or are breastfeeding, your employer must make sure that the kind of work you do and your working conditions will not put your health or your baby's health at risk. To get full benefit from this new legal protection, you must tell your employer in writing that you are pregnant or have recently given birth or are breastfeeding.

Your employer is required to take the following steps:

- Carry out a risk assessment at your workplace.

- Do all that is reasonable to remove or reduce the risks found.

131

THE TIMING OF YOUR RIGHTS AND BENEFITS IN PREGNANCY IS VERY COMPLICATED, SO USE THIS WEEKLY CHART AS A ROUGH GUIDE ONLY.

The week your baby is born.

If you haven't already told your employer when you are returning to work, you must do so by now, if you qualify for the extended 29-week maternity absence.

1 2 3 4 5 6 7 8 9 10 11 12 13 14 15 16 17 18 19 20 21 22 23 24 25 26 27 28 29

Claim child benefit as soon as you have registered your baby's birth and have the birth certificate.

If you qualify for a Maternity Payment from the Social Fund you must apply by now.

If you are taking maximum time off work, you must return to work before the end of this week.

- Give you information on the risks and the protective measures.

- If the risks still remain, your employer must alter your working conditions or hours of work, if it is reasonable to do so and would avoid the risk.

- If this is not possible or would not avoid the risk, your employer must offer you a suitable alternative job.

- If this is not possible your employer must suspend you on full pay for as long as is necessary to avoid the risks. If you have unreasonably refused alternative work offered by your employer you lose the right to full pay during your suspension.

- If you do night work and your doctor advises that you

should stop for health and safety reasons, you have the right to transfer to day work or be suspended on full pay. You must provide a medical certificate.

You cannot be dismissed because a health and safety risk means that you are unable to do all of your normal job. If you are worried or are refused any of these rights you should consult your trade union or get legal advice.

MATERNITY PAY AND BENEFITS

STATUTORY MATERNITY PAY (SMP)

What is it?
A weekly payment which is paid for a maximum of 18 weeks starting when you leave work to start your

maternity leave. **You can get it even if you do not plan to go back to work and you won't have to repay it.**

Who gets it?
You must have worked for the same employer for at least 26 weeks by the end of the 15th week before the week your baby is due (the 'qualifying week') and still be in your job in this week. (It doesn't matter if you are off work sick, or on holiday.) To work out which is the qualifying week look on the calendar for the Sunday before (or on) which your baby is due. *Not* counting that Sunday, count back 15 Sundays. The qualifying week begins on that Sunday. You could use the chart on pages 130–31 of this book.
You also need to be earning £62 a week or more on average in the 8 weeks (if you are paid weekly) or 2 months (if you are paid monthly) before the end of the qualifying week.
If you're not sure if you're

entitled to SMP, ask anyway. Your employer will work out whether or not you should get it.

How much is it?
For the first six weeks you get 90% of your average pay. (The average is calculated from the pay you actually received in the eight weeks or two months before the end of the qualifying week.) After that you get the basic rate of SMP which is £55.70 a week for up to 12 weeks.
You won't get SMP for any week that you work. So, if you qualify for only 14 weeks maternity leave and you return to work after the end of the 14th week, you will lose the last four weeks of your 18 weeks of SMP.

When is it paid?
It's up to you to decide when you want to start your maternity leave and pay. Week 11 before the birth is the earliest you can get SMP, but you can work

WOMEN WHO HAVE PAID NATIONAL INSURANCE

right up until the day your baby is due and you will not lose any SMP. The only exception to this rule is if you have a pregnancy-related illness in the last six weeks of your pregnancy. If this happens you will not be entitled to claim Statutory Sick Pay and will start receiving your maternity pay. If your illness is not pregnancy-related you can claim Statutory Sick Pay until your maternity leave and maternity pay start.

Your employer should pay your SMP weekly or monthly, in the same way as you are usually paid. They should deduct any tax and National Insurance contributions as necessary.

How do I get it?
Write to your employer at least 21 days before you stop work, telling them the date you are going on leave and asking for SMP. You must send them your maternity certificate (form MAT B1) which your GP or midwife will give you when you are about six months pregnant.

MATERNITY ALLOWANCE

What is it?
A weekly allowance for women who can't get SMP. It is paid for up to 18 weeks starting any time from 11 weeks before the week your baby is due. You can get Maternity Allowance if you are self-employed, if you gave up work, or if you changed jobs during your pregnancy.

Who gets it?
Women who can't get SMP but who have worked and paid full rate National Insurance contributions for at least 26 of the 66 weeks before the week in which the baby is due. If in doubt, claim. Your social security office (in Northern Ireland, the Incapacity Benefits Branch, Castle Court, Royal Avenue, Belfast BT1 1SB) will work out whether or not you can get the benefit.

How much is it?
There are two rates. The lower rate of £48.35 a week is paid to women who are either self-employed or unemployed in the qualifying week (the 15th week before the expected week of childbirth). A higher rate of £55.70 a week is paid to women who are employed in the qualifying week.

How do I claim?
(1) Fill in form MA1 (available from your social security office or your antenatal clinic) and send it to your local social security office (in Northern Ireland, the Incapacity Benefits Branch) along with
(2) your maternity certificate (form MAT B1) from your GP or midwife, and
(3) (if you are employed) form SMP1 which your employer will give you if you do not qualify for SMP. Send in form MA1 as soon as you can after you are 26 weeks pregnant. Don't put off sending it in because you are waiting for the MAT B1. You can send it later.
If you have not paid 26 weeks National Insurance contributions by the time you are 26 weeks pregnant, then you may decide to work later into your pregnancy. You should send off the MA1 form as soon as you have made 26 National Insurance contributions.

INCAPACITY BENEFIT

What is it?
A weekly benefit which is paid from six weeks before the birth until two weeks after the birth.

Who gets it?
If you can't get SMP or Maternity Allowance but have worked and paid National Insurance contributions in the last three years, you may be able to get this benefit.

How much is it?
£47.10 a week.

How do I claim?
Make a claim for Maternity Allowance using form MA1 (see above). If you're not entitled to Maternity Allowance, your social security office (in Northern Ireland the Incapacity Benefits Branch) will check to see if you can get any Incapacity Benefit. You don't need a sick note from your doctor, but do remember to send your maternity certificate, form MAT B1 with your claim. You should claim as soon as you can after you are 26 weeks pregnant.

USEFUL ORGANISATIONS

Some of these organisations are large. Many are small. Some offer advice or information face to face or over the telephone. Others concentrate on providing useful leaflets or books. Many have local branches or can put you in touch with local groups or a local contact.

Where there are separate addresses for the same or similar organisations in Scotland, Wales and Northern Ireland, these are given. If the UK is not covered by one or more organisations the area covered is indicated by 'E' – England, 'W' – Wales, 'NI' – Northern Ireland, 'S' – Scotland. If you live in Wales you can contact Health Information Wales 0800 665544 for information on local groups. If you live in Scotland and can't find the information you need in this section, contact the NHS Helpline in Scotland 0800 224488 where trained staff will answer your enquiries.

Organisations marked * produce publications. When you write for information it's important to remember to enclose a large stamped addressed envelope for a reply. Many organisations are run by volunteers and nearly all have a very tight budget.

SUPPORT AND INFORMATION

ACAS (Advisory, Conciliation and Arbitration Service)
(E, S & W)
Clifton House
83 Euston Road
London NW1 2RB
(0171) 396 5100
Advice on time off for antenatal care and on matters like unfair dismissal. For your nearest office, look in the phone book or ask at your local library or Citizens' Advice Bureau.*

Action on Pre-eclampsia (APEC)
31-33 College Road
Harrow
Middx HA1 1EJ
(0181) 406 3172
(01923) 266778 (24-hour helpline)
National charity offering support and information about pre-eclampsia via its helpline and newsletters. Provides a network of local contacts and groups. (Provides publication.)

Active Birth Centre
25 Bickerton Road
London N19 5JT
(0171) 561 9006
Promotes a holistic approach to childbirth. Antenatal and postnatal classes (fee payable). Publishes list of UK active birth teachers. (Provides publication.)

Association of Breastfeeding Mothers
PO Box 441
St Albans
Herts AL4 0AS
(0181) 778 4769 (Recorded information)
Telephone advice service for breastfeeding mothers and those wanting to breastfeed. Runs support groups (babies welcome). Help given to those wishing to set up a group in their area.*

Association for Improvements in the Maternity Services (AIMS)
40 Kingswood Avenue
London NW6 6LS
(0181) 960 5585
In Scotland:
40 Leamington Terrace
Edinburgh EH10 4JL
(0131) 229 6259
Voluntary pressure group which aims for improvements in maternity services. Support and advice about parents' rights, complaints procedures and choices within maternity care, including home birth.*

British Diabetic Association
10 Queen Anne Street
London W1M 0BD
(0171) 323 1531
In Northern Ireland:
John Gibson House
257 Lisburn Road
Belfast BT9 7EN
National charity offering information and support through a network of local groups to people with diabetes and their families.*
In Wales:
Plas Gwynt
Sophia Close
Cardiff CF1 9TD
(01222) 668276

Caesarean Support Network
55 Cooil Drive
Douglas
Isle of Man IN2 2HF
(01624) 661269 (Mon to Fri, after 6 pm and weekends)
Offers emotional support and practical advice to mothers who have had or may need a Caesarean delivery. Can put you in touch with a local mother who has undergone a Caesarean and understands the problems.*

Child
Charter House
43 St Leonards Road
Bexhill-on-Sea
E. Sussex TN40 1JA
(01424) 732361
Self-help organisation offering information and support to people coping with problems of infertility and childlessness. Telephone helplines for general problems and special helplines for specific problems like IVF, GIFT, ectopic pregnancies, miscarriages, stillbirths, endometriosis, polycystic ovaries and adoption. May be able to put you in touch with a local contact or group.*

Child Poverty Action Group (CPAG)
4th Floor
1-5 Bath Street
London EC1V 9PY
(0171) 253 3406
In Northern Ireland:
12 Queen Street
Londonderry BT48 7EG
(01504) 267777
Campaigns for children's rights and offers information on welfare benefits.

Citizens' Advice Bureau (CAB)
Information and advice on topics including benefits, maternity rights, debts, housing, consumer, employment and legal problems as well as family and personal difficulties. Have details of useful national and local organisations. Free and confidential. Opening times vary. Ask for the address at your local library or look in your phone book.*

Community Health Councils (CHCs)
(Local Health Councils in Scotland; local Health and Social Services Councils in Northern Ireland)
Represent the interests of consumers in the NHS services and your entitlements, and help you if you are having difficulties or wish to make a complaint. Have information on other local organisations. Look in the phone book under your health authority/health board/local Health and Social Services Council.

Equal Opportunities Commission
Overseas House
Quay Street
Manchester M3 3HN
(0161) 833 9244
In Northern Ireland:
Chamber of Commerce House
22 Great Victoria House
Belfast BT2 7BA
(01232) 242752
Information and advice on issues of discrimination and equal opportunities.*

Local health authorities
These have replaced Family Practitioner Committees. If you're new to an area they can give you a list of local doctors including those with a special interest in pregnancy and childbirth. If you have difficulty in finding a GP to take you on contact the LHA. Look in the phone book under the name of your local health authority/health board.
In Northern Ireland:
Contact your local Health and Social Services Board or the Central Services Agency for Health and Personal Social Services (CSA)
25 Adelaide Street
Belfast BT2 8FH
(01232) 324431

Family Welfare Association
501-505 Kingsland Road
London E8 4AU
(0171) 254 6251
National charity providing free social work services, e.g. counselling for relationship difficulties and advice on other problems. Provides grants for people in need throughout the UK.*

Independent Midwives Association
94 Auckland Road
Upper Norwood
London SE19 2DB
(0181) 406 3172
Free advice to women thinking about a home birth. Offers full care to women who book with them for home births. They also have their own birthing centres. Fees vary. Send an A5 SAE for information.*

Institute for Complementary Medicine
PO Box 194
London SE16 1QZ
(0171) 237 5165
(0171) 237 5175 (Fax)
Charity providing information on complementary medicine and referrals to qualified practitioners or helpful organisations. Please include SAE and loose stamps with written requests for information.*

La Leche League (Great Britain)
BM 3424
London WC1N 3XX
(0171) 242 1278 (24-hour answerphone)
Help and information for women wanting to breastfeed their babies, and personal counselling to mothers having problems in breastfeeding. Local groups hold friendly, informal discussions on breastfeeding, birth and parenthood.*

Labour Relations Agency (NI)
2-8 Gordon Street
Belfast BT1 2LG
(01232) 321442
Advice on maternity rights in Northern Ireland.*

Life
Life House
Newbold Terrace
Leamington Spa
Warwickshire CV32 4EA
(01926) 421587
(01926) 311511 (National hotline 9 am to 9 pm)
Charity offering information and advice on pregnancy, abortion, miscarriage, stillbirth and post-abortion counselling.

Local advice agencies
There may be a number of helpful local advice agencies in your district offering general advice on a range of topics, like benefits, debts and consumer problems, or specialising in one area such as law or housing. To find out what exists ask at your library or town hall.

Maternity Alliance
45 Beech Street
London EC2P 2LX
(0171) 588 8582 (Mon to Fri, 10 am to 1 pm)
Information on all aspects of maternity services, rights at work and benefits for families.*

Multiple Births Foundation
Queen Charlotte's and Chelsea Hospital
Goldhawk Road
London W6 0XG
(0181) 383 3519
Provides a range of services to families with twin, triplets and higher order births. (Provides publication.)

National Association for Maternal and Child Welfare
1st Floor
40-42 Osnaburgh Street
London NW1 3ND
(0171) 383 4115
Telephone advice on childcare and family life.*

National Childbirth Trust (NCT)
Alexandra House
Oldham Terrace
London W3 6NH
(0181) 992 8637
National charity with branches throughout the UK.
Runs antenatal classes giving information on labour and practice of relaxation, breathing, massage and active positions for labour and birth. Has breastfeeding counsellors who will help with feeding. Also offers postnatal support from other mothers and runs postnatal exercise classes in some areas. Provides information for parents with disabilities or medical conditions and puts them in touch with each other. Local branches.*

National Society for the Prevention of Cruelty to Children (NSPCC)
42 Curtain Road
London EC2A 3NH
(0171) 825 2500
0800 800500 Child Protection Helpline
In Northern Ireland:
Jenny Mount Court
North Derby Street
Belfast BT15 3HN
(01232) 351135
In Wales:
9 Brindley Road
Cardiff CF1 7TX
(01222) 371080
Aims to prevent all forms of child abuse. If you're in need of help or know of anyone who needs help, look in the phone book for your nearest NSPCC office.*

**National Health Information Service (England)
Health Information Wales/Cyswllt Iechyd Cymru**
0800 665544 (Freephone, 10 am to 5 pm, minicom available)
A confidential information service on health service matters and self-help groups.

NHS Helpline in Scotland
0800 224488
Provides comprehensive information about health services and the NHS in Scotland. Covers health education, patient rights, waiting times, GPs, pharmacists, opticians, community services and hospital services. Free leaflets on a wide range of health topics are also available and calls are fee and confidential.*

Northern Ireland Housing Executive
2 Adelaide Street
Belfast BT2 8PB
(01232) 240588
Offers advice and information on all aspects of housing for Northern Ireland.

Patients' Association
PO Box 935
Harrow
Middx HA1 3YJ
(0181) 423 8999
Advice service for patients who have difficulties with their doctor.*

Public libraries
Useful starting points for finding out addresses of national and local organisations. Librarians are usually helpful in producing information or in pointing you in the right direction.

Relate: Marriage Guidance
Herbert Gray College
Little Church Street
Rugby CV21 3AP
(01788) 573241
In Northern Ireland:
Northern Ireland Marriage Guidance Council (Relate)
76 Dublin Road
Belfast BT2 7HP
(01232) 323454
Confidential counselling on relationship problems of any kind. Look in the phone book for your local branch under 'Relate' or 'Marriage Guidance' or contact one of the above addresses.*

Shelter, the National Campaign for the Homeless
88 Old Street
London EC1V 9HU
(0171) 505 2000
0800 446441 (Freephone)
In Northern Ireland:
165 University Street
Belfast BT7 1HR
(01232) 247752
In Wales:
Shelter Wales/Shelter Cymru
25 Walter Road
Swansea
West Glamorgan SA1 5NN
(01792) 469400
0800 802010 (Mon to Fri, 2 pm to 7 pm)
Information and advice on housing matters, including tenants' rights, welfare rights, how to claim improvement grants, etc.
If you have housing difficulties, seek advice as soon as possible. Accommodation law is very complex and you could be jeopardising your chances of finding a suitable home. Contact for details of your local Shelter Housing Aid Centre.*

Social Security: Freeline
For general advice on all social security benefits, pensions and National Insurance including maternity benefits and Income Support, phone Freeline Social Security on 0800 666555 between 9 am and 4.30 pm on weekdays, and between 9 am and 1 pm on Saturday mornings. Calls are free. There is an answerphone service out of hours.
Advice in Urdu or Punjabi:
Phone Freeline
0800 289188 between 9 am and 4 pm weekdays.
For Punjabi only telephone Freeline 0800 521360 during the same hours.

For general advice on all social security benefits, pensions and National Insurance, including maternity benefits, Income Support and Income-based Jobseeker's Allowance, telephone, write or call in to your local social security office. The address will be in the phone book under 'Social Security'. Hours are usually 9.30 am to 3.30 pm. In busy offices there may be a very long wait if you call in.

Social services

A social worker at your local social services area office will give you information on topics including benefits, housing, financial difficulties, employment, relationship problems, childcare and useful organisations. Look up social services in the phone book under the name of your local authority/local Health and Social Services Board or ask at your local library. Phone, write or call in. There may also be a social worker based at the hospital to whom you could talk, either during your antenatal care or when you or your baby are in hospital. Ask your midwife or other hospital staff to put you in contact.

Twins and Multiple Births Association (TAMBA)

PO Box 30
Little Sutton
S. Wirral L66 1TH
(0151) 348 0020 (9 am to 2 pm; answerphone)
TAMBA Twinline (Helpline)
(01732) 868000 (6 pm to 11 pm weekdays; 8 am to 11 pm weekends)
Self-help organisation to encourage and support parents of twins, triplets or more. Will put parents in touch with local support groups, or specialist groups for parents of triplets or more, parents of children with special needs or bereaved parents, if appropriate.*

Women's Aid Federation

PO Box 391
Bristol BS99 7WS
(01345) 023 468
In Northern Ireland:
Women's Aid Federation
129 University Street
Belfast BT7 1HP
(01232) 249041
In Scotland:
Scottish Women's Aid
12 Torphichen Street
Edinburgh EH3 8JQ
(0131) 221 0401 (10 am to 1 pm)
(0131) 221 0402 (Fax)
In Wales:
Welsh Women's Aid
38-48 Crwys Road
Cardiff CF2 4NN
(01222) 390874/878
Advice, support and accommodation to women who have been abused mentally, physically or sexually, and their children. Local groups.*

COPING ALONE

Gingerbread

16-17 Clerkenwell Close
London EC1R 0AA
(0171) 336 8184 Mon to Fri 11 am-4 pm
In Northern Ireland:
Gingerbread Northern Ireland
169 University Street
Belfast BT7 1HR
(01232) 231417
In Wales:
Gingerbread Wales:
Room 1
Mansel House
99 Mansel Street
Swansea SA1 5UE
(01792) 648728 (Answerphone)
Self-help associations for one-parent families. A network of local groups offers mutual support, friendship, information, advice and practical help. Do get in touch if you are pregnant and on your own.*

MAMA (Meet-a-mum Association)

26 Avenue Road
South Norwood
London SE25 4DX
(0181) 771 5595
In Wales:
Room 1
Mansel House
99 Mansel Street
Swansea SA1 5UE
Support for mothers suffering from postnatal depression or who feel lonely and isolated looking after a child at home. Will try to put you in touch with another mother who has experienced similar problems, or with a group of mothers locally, or help you to find ways of meeting people.*

National Council for One Parent Families (E, W & NI)

255 Kentish Town Road
London NW5 2LX
(0171) 267 1361 (not Wednesdays)
In Scotland:
One Parent Families Scotland
13 Gayfield Square
Edinburgh EH1 3NX
(0131) 556 3899
Information on benefits and employment rights in pregnancy, social security, taxation, housing problems and maintenance.*

Parents Advice Centre (NI)

Franklin House
12 Brunswick Street
Belfast BT2 7GE
(01232) 238800
(Answerphone after hours with details and contact numbers)
A confidential service offering support and guidance to parents under stress.

Parents Anonymous

6-9 Manor Gardens
London N7 6LA
(0171) 263 8918 (Answerphone)
Telephone helpline run by volunteers for parents under stress who feel they can't cope or might abuse their children.

LOSS AND BEREAVEMENT

(See also 'Child' under Support and information.)

Compassionate Friends

53 North Street
Bristol BS3 1EN
(0117) 953 9639
An organisation of and for bereaved parents. Advice and support. Local groups.*

Foundation for the Study of Infant Deaths (Cot Death Research and Support)

(E, W & NI)
14 Halkin Street
London SW1X 7DP
(0171) 235 0965
In Northern Ireland:
Friends of the Foundation for the Study of Infant Deaths
7 Glenaan Avenue
Belfast BT17 9AT
(01232) 622688 (Answerphone)
Support and information for parents bereaved by a sudden infant death, and support with any subsequent babies. Can put parents in touch with local support groups of other parents who have also suffered bereavement. Produce infant care guidance card including symptoms of serious illness to watch out for in babies.*

Miscarriage Association

c/o Clayton Hospital
Northgate
Wakefield
W. Yorks WF1 3JS
(01924) 200799
Information, advice and support for women who have had, or who are having, a miscarriage. Local contacts and groups.*

SATFA (Support Around Termination for Abnormality) (E, W & NI)

73 Charlotte Street
London W1P 1LB
(0171) 631 0285 (Helpline)
Registered charity offering support and information to parents who are concerned about antenatal testing, or are faced with the decision of whether to terminate a pregnancy following the diagnosis of abnormality in their unborn baby. Ongoing support given to parents who decide to terminate pregnancy. Network of local contacts and groups sharing similar experiences.

Stillbirth and Neonatal Death Society (SANDS)

28 Portland Place
London W1N 4DE
(0171) 436 5881
Support and information with a national network of groups for bereaved parents.*

ILLNESS AND DISABILITY

Action for Sick Children (E)

Argyle House
29-31 Euston Road
London NW1 2SD
(0171) 833 2041 (9 am to 5 pm; recorded message out of hours)
In Scotland:
Action for Sick Children
15 Smith's Place
Edinburgh EH6 8HT
(0131) 553 6553 (Answerphone)
In Wales:
Association for the Welfare of Children in Hospital (AWCH)
31 Penyrheol Drive
Sketty
Swansea
(01792) 205227
In Northern Ireland:
AWCH
Bryson House
28 Bedford Street
Belfast BT2 7FE
(01232) 799215 (after 6 pm)
Advice and support for families with sick children. Helps them make use of the health service. Telephone advice. There may be a local group you can join.*

BLISS

17-21 Emerald Street
London WC1N 3QL
(0171) 831 9393
Parent support network providing emotional and practical support to the families of babies who need intensive or special care. Local groups.*

Contact a Family

170 Tottenham Court Road
London W1P 0HA
(0171) 383 3555
National charity offering information, advice and support to parents of children with special needs and disabilities. Links parents to local support groups for general support or to nationally run groups or, in the case of rare disorder, to individuals in similar circumstances.*

Council for Disabled Children

Wakley Street
London EC1V 7QE
(0171) 843 6061
Information for parents and details of organisations offering help with particular disbilities.*

Disabled Living Centre (NI)

Musgrave Park Hospital
Stockman's Lane
Belfast BT9 7JB
(01232) 669501 ext 2708
Information and advice on all aspects of disability, especially equipment and dealing with living problems. Referral to other organisations for adults and children with disabilities.

Disability Action (NI)

2 Annadale Avenue
Belfast BT7 3JH
(01232) 491011
Provides information and advice on physical disability and local organisations.

Disability Information Trust

Mary Marlborough Centre
Nuffield Orthopaedic Centre
Windmill Road
Headington
Oxford OX3 7LD
(01865) 227592 (Answerphone)
Assesses and tests equipment for people with disabilities. Publishes information in series Equipment for Disabled People.

Genetic Interest Group (GIG)

Farringdon Point
29-35 Farringdon Road
London EC1M 3JB
(0171) 430 0090
Umbrella body for support groups working with those affected by specific genetic disorders. Provides information for individuals at risk and their families about services available within the NHS and elsewhere. Can put you in touch with the relevant support group.

Northern Ireland Mother and Baby Appeal (NIMBA)

(NI)
15 Stranmillis Road
Belfast BT9 5AF
(01232) 667166
A local charity offering support and advice to parents of premature, ill or disabled babies who need intensive or special care. A parents' support network is available throughout Northern Ireland.

SPECIALISED ORGANISATIONS

Association of Parents of Vaccine Damaged Children

78 Campden Road
Shipston-on-Stour
Warwickshire CV36 4DH
(01608) 661595
Advises parents on claiming vaccine damage payment.

Association for Spina Bifida and Hydrocephalus (ASBAH)

(E & W)
ASBAH House
42 Park Road
Peterborough PE1 2UQ
(01733) 555988
In Scotland:
Scottish Spina Bifida Association
190 Queensferry Road
Edinburgh EH4 2BW
(0131) 332 0743
In Northern Ireland:
Northern Ireland Spina Bifida and Hydrocephalus Association
Graham House
Knockbracken Healthcare Park
Saintfield Road
Belfast BT8 8BH
(01232) 798878
(01232) 797071 (Fax)
Information, advice, counselling and support for parents. Local support groups.*

Cleft Lip and Palate Association (CLAPA)

134 Buckingham Palace Road
London SW1W 9SA
(0121) 824 8110
Voluntary organisation of parents and professionals offering support to families of babies born with cleft lip and/or palate. Feeding equipment available. Local groups.*

Cystic Fibrosis Trust

11 London Road
Bromley BR1 1BY
(0181) 464 7211
In Northern Ireland:
Cystic Fibrosis Trust in Northern Ireland
20 Bryansburn Road
Bangor
Co Down BT20 3SB
(01247) 272781 (Answerphone)
In Wales:
Cystic Fibrosis Trust in Wales
WVA
Llys Ifor
Crescent Road
Caerphilly CF83 1XL
(01222) 852751
Information and support for parents of children with cystic fibrosis and for people worried about the possibility of passing on the illness. Local groups.*

Down's Syndrome Association (E & W)

155 Mitcham Road
Tooting
London SW17 9PG
(0181) 682 4001
In Scotland:
Scottish Down's Syndrome Association
158-160 Balgreen Road
Edinburgh EH11 3AU
(0131) 313 4225
In Northern Ireland:
Down's Syndrome Association
Graham House
Knockbracken Healthcare Park
Saintfield Road
Belfast BT8 8BH
(01232) 704606
Information, advice, counselling and support for parents of children with Down's syndrome. Local groups. 24-hour helpline.*

Haemophilia Society

Chesterfield House
385 Euston Road
London NW3 3AU
(0171) 380 0600
In Northern Ireland:
Society House
6 Kilcoole Park
Belfast BT14 8LB
(01232) 729559
Information, advice and practical help for families affected by haemophilia. Some local groups.*

Jennifer Trust for Spinal Muscular Atrophy

11 Ash Tree Close
Wellesbourne
Warwickshire CV35 9SA
(01789) 842377 (9 am to 3 pm; answerphone)
Self-help group offering information and support to parents of children with the disease. Can put you in touch with other parents. Equipment on loan.*

MENCAP (Royal Society for Mentally Handicapped Children and Adults)

(E, W & NI)
MENCAP National Centre
123 Golden Lane
London EC1Y 0RT
(0171) 454 0454
In Scotland:
ENABLE (S)
6th Floor
7 Buchanan Street
Glasgow G1 3HL
(0141) 226 4541
In Northern Ireland:
MENCAP in Northern Ireland
4 Annadale Avenue
Belfast BT7 3JH
(01232) 691351
In Wales:
MENCAP in Wales
31 Lambourne Crescent
Cardiff Business Park
Llanishen
Cardiff CF4 5GG
(01222) 747 588
Information, support and advice for parents of children with learning disabilities. Local groups.*

Meningitis Research Foundation
13 High Street
Thornbury
Bristol BS12 2AE
(01454) 413344
In Northern Ireland:
71 Botanic Avenue
Belfast BT7 1JL
(01232) 321283
In Scotland:
133 Guilmore Place
Edinburgh EH3 9TP
(0131) 228 3324
(01454) 413344 (24-hour national helpline)
Offers counselling for parents whose children have died from meningitis and gives support to people with loved ones in hospital or at home.*

Muscular Dystrophy Group of Great Britain and Northern Ireland
7-11 Prescott Place
London SW4 6BS
(0171) 720 8055
Information, advice and support for families affected by muscular dystrophy.*

National Society for Phenylketonuria and Allied Disorders
7 Southfield Close
Willen
Milton Keynes MK15 9LL
(01908) 691653
(Answerphone)
Self-help organisation offering information and support to families affected by the disorder. Newsletter.*

Northern Ireland Council for Orthopaedic Development (NICOD)
Malcolm Sinclair House
31 Ulsterville Avenue
Belfast BT9 7AS
(01232) 666188
Offers advice and support to parents of children with cerebral palsy.*

REACH (The Association for Children with Hand or Arm Deficiency)
12 Wilson Way
Earls Barton
North Hampshire NN6 0NZ
(01604) 811041
(Answerphone)
Information and support to parents of children with hand or arm problems. Can put you in touch with individual families in a similar situation or local groups.*

SENSE (National Deaf-Blind and Rubella Association)
11-13 Clifton Terrace
Finsbury Park
London N4 3SR
(0171) 272 7774
In Northern Ireland:
The Resource Centre
Knockbracken Healthcare Park
Saintfield Road
Belfast BT8 8BH
(01232) 705858
Information, advice and support for families of deaf-blind and rubella-handicapped children.*
In Wales:
SENSE Cymru
Shand House
20 Newport Road
Cardiff CF2 1YB

Sickle Cell Society
54 Station Road
Harlesden
London NW10 4UA
(0181) 961 7795/8346
Information, advice and counselling on sickle cell disorders.*
In Wales:
Sickle Cell and Thalassaemia Centre
Butetown Health Centre
Loudoun Square
Butetown
Cardiff
(01222) 471055

Society for Mucopolysaccharide Diseases
55 Hill Avenue
Amersham
Buckinghamshire HP6 5BX
(01494) 434156/762789
Information and support to families of children affected by this and related disorders. Local groups.*

SCOPE
12 Park Crescent
London W1N 4EQ
(0171) 636 5020
(0800) 626216 (E and W helpline Mon-Sat 11 am to 9 pm; 2 pm to 6 pm Sun)
In Wales:
3 Links Court
Links Business Park
St Mellons
Cardiff CF3 0SP
(01222) 797706
Offers advice and support to parents of children with cerebral palsy.*

Tay Sachs and Allied Diseases Association
c/o Postgraduate and Research Centre
Royal Manchester Children's Hospital
Pendlebury
Manchester M27 4HA
(0161) 794 4696 ext 2384
(Answerphone)
Screening for carrier status before and during pregnancy. Information, counselling and practical support to families affected by these disorders.*

Toxoplasmosis Trust
Room 26
61-71 Collier Street
London N1 9BE
(0171) 713 0599
Information, advice and counselling for pregnant women with toxoplasmosis, parents of infected children and others with toxoplasmosis.*

The UK Thalassaemia Society
19 The Broadway
Southgate Circus
London N14 6PH
(0181) 882 0011
Information, advice and support for families affected by thalassaemia and for possible carriers.*

CHILDCARE

Daycare Trust/National Childcare Campaign
4 Wild Court
London WC2B 4AU
(0171) 405 5617
Information and advice on obtaining suitable forms of childcare and on setting up day care.*

National Childminding Association (E & W)
8 Masons Hill
Bromley BR2 9EY
(0181) 464 6164
In Scotland:
Scottish Childminding Association
Room 7
Stirling Business Centre
Stirling FK8 2DZ
(01786) 445377
In Northern Ireland:
Northern Ireland Childminding Association
17A Court Street
Newtownards
Co Down BT23 3NX
(01247) 811015
Associations for childminders, childcare workers, parents and others who are interested in day care and wish to improve it.*

Northern Ireland Pre-School Playgroups Association (NIPPA) (NI)
Unit 3
Enterprise House
Boucher Crescent
Belfast BT12 6HU
(01232) 662825
A voluntary association of mother and toddler groups, playgroups and families of the under-5s who attend them. Provides help and support through a network covering Northern Ireland.

Working for Childcare
77 Holloway Road
London N7 8JZ
(0171) 700 0281
Advice and information for employers, trade unions and parents on developing childcare at work.

FAMILY PLANNING

Brook Advisory Centres (E, S & NI)
165 Gray's Inn Road
London WC1X 8UD
(0171) 713 9000
Advice and practical help with contraception and pregnancy testing, advice on unplanned pregnancies and sexual counselling for young men and women. Free and confidential. For your nearest centre look in the local phone book or contact Brook Central Office.*

Family Planning Association
2-12 Pentonville Road
London NW1 9FP
(0171) 837 5432
In Northern Ireland:
113 University Street
Belfast BT7 1HP
(01232) 325488
In Wales:
4 Museum Place
Cardiff CF1 3BG
(01222) 342766
Information on all aspects of family planning and methods of contraception.*

Marie Stopes Clinic
Marie Stopes House
108 Whitfield Street
London W1P 6BE
(0171) 388 0662
Registered charity providing family planning, women's health check-ups, male and female sterilisation, pregnancy testing, advice on unplanned pregnancies and sexual counselling for men and women. You don't need to be referred by your doctor, but you do need to book an appointment. A charge is made to cover costs. For centres in Manchester and Leeds look in the local phone book.*

ALCOHOL

Alcohol Concern
Waterbridge House
32-36 Loman Street
London SE1 0EE
(0171) 928 7377
In Wales:
Welsh Drug and Alcohol Unit
4th Floor
St David's House
Woodstreet
Cardiff CF1 2ER
(01222) 667766
In Scotland:
Scottish National Alcohol Charity
2nd Floor
166 Buchanan Street
Glasgow G1 2NH
(0141) 333 9677
Information on alcohol problems, what types of services exist and where you can get help locally.*

Alcoholics Anonymous (AA) (E, S & W)
AA General Service Office
PO Box 1
Stonebow House
Stonebow
York YO1 2NJ
(01904) 644026
Network of independent self-help groups whose members encourage each other to stop drinking and to stay off drink. First names only are used to preserve anonymity. For your nearest group look in the phone book or contact the AA General Service Office.*

Drinkline
Alcohol Helpline
(0345) 320202

Dunlewey Substance Advice Centre (NI)
226 Stewartstown Road
Belfast BT7 0LB
(01232) 611162
Offers help and personal counselling on alcohol, drug and solvent abuse. Employment support programme.

Northern Ireland Community Addiction Service Ltd (NICAS) (NI)
40 Elmwood Avenue
Belfast BT9 6AZ
(01232) 664434
Provides counselling, treatment, education, information and training on dealing with alcohol and drug addiction.

Northlands (NI)
13 Pump Street
Londonderry BT48 6JG
(01504) 263356
Gives advice, information and counselling for those with alcohol or other drug-related problems.

SMOKING

Quitline
0800 00 22 00
Quitline in Wales
(0345) 697500
Advice on stopping smoking and details of local stop smoking support services. Phone between 9.30 am and 5.30 pm on weekdays. Recorded advice available at other times. If you prefer to write for information:

Quit*
Victory House
170 Tottenham Court Road
London W1P 0HA
(0171) 388 5775

Ulster Cancer Foundation
40 Eglantine Avenue
Belfast BT9 6DX
(01232) 663281/2/3
Carries out cancer research and education programmes in Northern Ireland. Also provides information on the dangers of smoking and provides advice and support to smokers who want to quit.

ADDICTIVE DRUGS

(See also 'Dunlewey Substance Advice Centre' 'Northlands' and 'NICAS' under Alcohol)

Drugaid Cardiff (W)
1 Neville Street
Cardiff CF1 8LP
Meetings every Wednesday from 6.30 pm to 9 pm. If you need advice outside of meetings, call Freephone 0800 776600 (English) or 0800 371141 (Welsh).

Narcotics Anonymous (UK service)
202 City Road
London EC1V 2PH
(0171) 251 4007
(0171) 730 0009 (Helpline)
Self-help organisation whose members help each other to stay clear of drugs. Phone between 12 pm and 8 pm for information and the address of your local group. Some groups have a crèche.

SCODA (The Standing Conference on Drug Abuse)
(E, NI & W)
Waterbridge House
32-36 Loman Street
London SE1 0EE
(0171) 928 9500
In Scotland:
Scottish Drug Forum
Shaftsbury House
5 Waterloo Street
Glasgow G2 6AY
(0141) 221 1175
Information on local treatment and services for drug users, family and friends.*

In England you can also ask the operator for Freefone Drug Problems which will give you a contact number for your local area. Or you can call the National Drugs Helpline on Freephone 0800 776600. In Wales you can also call Freephone 0800 371141 (Welsh).

HIV AND AIDS

Aids Helpline (NI)
0800 137437 (7 pm to 10 pm weekdays; 2 pm to 5 pm Saturday)

Body Positive
51B Philbeach Gardens
London SW5 9EB
(0171) 373 9124 (Helpline 7 pm to 10 pm)
Counselling services and support for women affected by HIV and AIDS, their family, partners and friends. For address and phone number of your local group phone the National AIDS Helpline or the above number.

National AIDS Helpline
0800 567123
Calls are confidential, free and available 24 hours a day. There is a Minicom on 0800 521361 for people who are deaf or hard of hearing.
Information in other languages:
Arabic - 0800 282447
(6 pm to 10 pm on Thursday);
Bengali - 0800 371132
(6 pm to 10 pm on Tuesday);
Cantonese - 0800 282446
(6 pm to 10 pm on Monday);
Gujarati - 0800 371134
(6 pm to 10 pm on Wednesday);
Hindi - 0800 371136
(6 pm to 10 pm on Wednesday);
Punjabi - 0800 371133
(6 pm to 10 pm on Wednesday);
Urdu - 0800 371135
(6 pm to 10 pm on Wednesday);
Welsh - 0800 371131
(10 am to 2 am daily). Leaflets can be ordered in all these languages.*

Positively Women
347-349 City Road
London EC1V 1LR
(0171) 713 0222 Mon to Fri 10 am to 4.30 pm, Mon and Thurs 5pm to 9 pm (Helpline)
(0171) 713 0444 (Admin)
Information and practical and emotional support for women with a positive HIV diagnosis or who have ARC or AIDS, including women who are pregnant or who have children. Support group.*

SUPPORT FOR STRESS OR DEPRESSION

Association for Post-Natal Illness (APNI)
25 Jerdan Place
London SW6 1BE
(0171) 386 0868
Network of telephone and postal volunteers who have suffered from postnatal illness and offer information, support and encouragement on a one-to-one basis. Send for information pack.

CRY-SIS
(E, W & NI)
BM CRY-SIS
London WC1N 3XX
(0171) 404 5011
Help and support for parents whose children cry excessively, have a sleep problem or have temper tantrums and other behaviour difficulties. Local voluntary counsellors who have experienced the same difficulties.*

Parentline
(E, S, W & NI)
Endway House
The Endway
Hadleigh
Essex SS7 2AN
(01702) 554782
(01702) 559900
(Helpline, 9 am to 9 pm weekdays, 2 pm to 6 pm Saturday)
A national helpline for anyone parenting a child who may need support, information or guidance.